Book Description

Unlock your body's potential for flexibility and balance as you age.

Do your joints creak and pop more than they used to?

Do you struggle with stiffness, limited mobility, or poor balance?

Do you want to carry on with your daily activities without worrying about stiffness getting in the way?

Aging doesn't mean discomfort is inevitable. With simple daily stretching, you can gain flexibility, balance, and pain relief for an improved quality of life. This comprehensive guide shares stretching routines specifically designed for seniors. Stretching only a few minutes a day can make a significant difference in how you feel. Regular senior stretches have benefits you will notice right away.

In this book, you will:

- Improve range of motion and limber up stiff, tight muscles, and target critical areas like your back, hips, legs, neck, shoulders, and core.

- Build strength to make daily tasks easier.

- Reduce the risk of falls or injury with better balance and coordination.

- Manage chronic pain and arthritis. Relieve joint pain in your knees, back, hands, and more through gentle movements.

- Adapt exercises to your current fitness level. Do them standing, sitting, or lying down - no special equipment is needed.

- Warm-up and cool down properly before and after exercise. This helps maximize benefits and prevent injury.

- Incorporate yoga poses and Pilates techniques modified for seniors. Increase flexibility, balance, and inner calm.

- Develop core stability for better posture and everyday functioning. Strengthen your back and abdominal muscles.

- Make stretching a consistent habit. Stay motivated with goal-setting, self-care tips, and finding a community.

- Address safety concerns like osteoporosis. Learn modifications to avoid harm.

You're never too old to feel young again. With the proper guidance, seniors can overcome physical limitations and rediscover their body's potential. This book provides the special techniques and care you need. This stretching guide empowers seniors to take charge of their health, featuring step-by-step instructions and clear illustrations. Follow customized routines that target areas prone to stiffness as you age. The result is relief from persistent aches, easier movement, improved balance and coordination, and an overall sense of rejuvenation.

So click on the "Add to Cart" button now and make small adjustments for big changes in comfort, mobility, and independence.

Stretching for Seniors

Keep Your Mind and Body Young with Daily Range of Motion Stretches

Table of Contents

Introduction

As you age, staying active and mobile becomes imperative for keeping your health and independence. Gentle stretching is one of the easiest yet most beneficial exercises for seniors. This book will teach you stretching routines tailored for the elderly and the substantial physical and mental benefits they offer.

The book discusses why flexibility should be prioritized as you age and how regular stretching enhances mobility and balance. You'll learn proper techniques to protect your body while maximizing results. Only a few minutes of stretching each day can dramatically improve your comfort and range of motion.

The book explains the natural age-related changes to your muscles, joints, and bones. It addresses common senior conditions like arthritis, osteoporosis, and circulation issues and how stretching helps manage them. You'll understand why staying flexible through activity is essential to maintaining mobility and vitality in your later years.

Moreover, the book covers the importance of warming up and cooling down before and after stretching and provides routines to get your blood flowing safely. Step-by-step instructions for upper and lower body stretches teach you to gently target your arms, legs, back, hips, neck, and core. The book includes modifications for standing and seated positions.

Balance and stability will decline with age, leading to increased fall risk. The book shares exercises and techniques to improve balance and confidence in seniors. Also, it discusses how to make balance activities safer.

Gentle yoga and Pilates are awesome complementary activities to build core strength and flexibility. The book provides senior-friendly beginner poses and mat exercises to increase stretching benefits.

Managing common aches and pains through targeted stretching is also covered. The book shares the most effective stretches to alleviate pain in the lower back, knees, hips, neck, and other frequently painful areas. Always consult a doctor before starting a new exercise.

No routine will stick without motivation. So, tips to help you maintain a consistent stretching habit are included. The book offers advice on goal-setting, finding stretch buddies, and making flexibility a daily priority.

By the conclusion, you'll understand why gentle stretching should be part of every senior's daily wellness routine. Further resources are included in this book to continue your flexibility journey. This book will motivate you to improve your physical and mental health with simple stretching.

Chapter 1: Introduction to Senior Stretching

Aging brings natural changes to the body. But accompanied by the gifts of wisdom and experience comes decreased physical flexibility and mobility. However, seniors can maintain and improve flexibility through stretching exercises, helping them stay active and enjoy life fully. This chapter explores the importance and benefits of senior stretching and covers safety factors to consider. While growing older transforms the body, stretching helps seniors make the most of their later years. Simple exercises support physical health and an engaged lifestyle.

The Importance of Flexibility for Seniors

Flexibility refers to the muscles and joints' ability to move freely through their range of motion. Your joints, like knees and hips, are meant to bend and straighten fully. Flexible muscles stretch without feeling tight or strained.

As you age, your muscles and joints stiffen without regular stretching. Muscles shorten, tendons get less flexible, and joints develop creaky calcium deposits and arthritis.

This loss of mobility makes everyday activities harder - for instance, looking over your shoulder or bending over becomes tricky. Poor posture, muscle imbalance, and tension creep up, too, and you lose range of motion bit by bit. Gradually, the limited flexibility impacts your active life and independence.

However, incorporating flexibility exercises, like stretching, can significantly slow this decline. Stretching keeps your muscles elongated and joints mobile.

Maintaining flexibility provides essential benefits:

1. Preserving Your Independence

One of the most important reasons for seniors to stay flexible is maintaining independence in daily living. The easier it is to move without limitation or pain, the longer you can perform routine activities without assistance.

Consider a few examples. Turning your head helps you safely back up your car and merge into traffic or parallel park. Adequate shoulder flexibility enables you to reach across your body to buckle a seatbelt. The ability to bend down preserves your ability to tie shoes or pick up dropped items.

Around the home, flexibility allows you to reach high shelves or cabinets comfortably. It helps when stepping into a bathtub or pulling clothes out of the washer. Yard work, like gardening or lawn care, requires free joint movement. The list goes on and on.

Remaining flexible to complete day-to-day tasks without help maintains self-reliance and dignity. Stretching programs combined with light resistance exercises give seniors the mobility to live life on their own terms.

2. Injury Prevention

Tense, stiff muscles and joints are more prone to strains, sprains, and tears because inflexible tissues can't handle sudden movements or absorb forces. Picture a stiff rubber band being pulled versus a loose, pliable one. The tight band would be more likely to snap when tugged.

For seniors, injuries due to falling are a significant concern. Limited mobility and poor balance further increase the risks. However, improving overall flexibility bolsters stability and helps avoid falls.

A full range of motion enhances your ability to catch yourself if you lose your balance. Flexible muscles coordinate quicker to prevent you from falling. They help absorb the impact of a fall, preventing serious injury. The protective benefits of flexibility against falls and mobility-related injuries are far-reaching.

Having flexibility safeguards against problems like arthritis and back pain. Tight muscles pull joints out of alignment, causing excessive strain and wear. A limited range of motion forces joints to compress rather than smoothly glide. By maintaining flexibility, joints can move through their natural arcs without added pressure, reducing inflammation and damage.

3. Improved Posture

Posture declines with age as muscles weaken and imbalances set in. Forward head position, rounded shoulders, and excessive kyphosis (upper back curvature) are common. Limited flexibility in the hips, hamstrings, chest, and abdominals contributes heavily to poor posture.

Regular stretching can help return muscles to their ideal lengths and balance tightness. For example, opening up tight chest muscles through the doorway stretches and combats rounded shoulders, gentle backbends counteract kyphosis, and flexibility exercises build core strength to support better posture.

Seniors experience less pain, move more efficiently, and have an easier time breathing with improved posture. Aligning the spine properly through flexibility work minimizes pain-causing joint pressure. Given how detrimental posture problems can become, stretching is protective.

4. Enhanced Quality of Life

Being flexible directly relates to your ability to participate in activities for personal fulfillment. Hobbies like gardening, golfing, dancing, and exercising require free joint mobility. Caring for grandchildren demands agility to keep up with youngster's demands. Even everyday joys like traveling and volunteering rely on flexibility.

Think of activities you love but struggle with presently. Maybe knee stiffness makes walking the dog difficult, or shoulder tightness hinders your golf swing. Perhaps lower back tightness prevents you from bending over in the garden. Improving flexibility could help you reclaim these joys.

Flexibility promotes better sleep, which greatly affects mood and vitality. Relieving muscle tension through stretching enables seniors to sleep comfortably and rest deeply. With enhanced flexibility, everyday movements cause less strain, allowing energy reserves to be channeled into what matters most.

When mobility limitations force seniors to give up activities that bring happiness, it directly diminishes their quality of life. Dedicated stretching can keep you moving freely and engaging in what sets your soul on fire.

Benefits of Regular Stretching

Strengthening your body through stretching provides immense benefits for seniors physically and mentally. These benefits include:

1. Increased Range of Motion

As you age, your tendons, ligaments, and muscles naturally lose elasticity and shorten, and joints accumulate calcium deposits. These changes restrict your range of motion, making everyday movements like bending, looking over your shoulder, and getting in and out of a car more challenging. Hence, limited mobility threatens independence.

However, regular stretching helps counteract this process by re-lengthening muscles and keeping joints supple. Stretching helps "open up" areas that have gotten tight and limited in motion. Simple stretches improve the mobility of major joints like the shoulders, hips, neck, and lower back.

For example, a sitting hamstring stretch lengthens the muscles in the back of the thigh. This simple stretch allows you to extend your leg further, making getting in and out of the car easier. Arm-across-chest stretches open up tight shoulder muscles, making reaching behind you easier.

2. Relief from Aches and Pains

As you experience normal age-related stiffening, overuse and improper movements can lead to chronic tension and discomfort. Limited mobility stresses joints by forcing them into awkward positions. These factors contribute to widespread pain.

However, stretching helps alleviate these issues in several key ways. First, regular stretching reduces muscle stiffness, pulling your body out of alignment and causing pain. Stretching lengthens muscles that are abnormally shortened due to disuse or repetitive strain. It releases unnecessary tension.

For example, tight hip flexor muscles often cause lower back discomfort. Stretching the hip flexors realigns the hips and pelvis, releasing pressure. Tight chest muscles lead to neck and shoulder discomfort, so stretching the pectoral muscles allows the shoulders to retract.

Stretching lubricates joints, allowing them to move smoothly rather than stiffly grinding, reducing inflammation and causing pain. Drinking water before and after stretching helps hydrate tissues for better shock absorption.

3. Better Circulation

Stretching delivers benefits beneath the skin by enhancing circulation. Moving the muscles and joints through their range of motion increases blood flow throughout the body. The effects are two-fold:

First, increased blood supply delivers oxygen and nutrients to the muscles and tissues. It aids recovery from exercise and improves the health of muscles, connective tissue, and skin. Warm, nutrient-rich blood also helps joints stay lubricated and nourished.

Second, enhanced circulation reduces the risk of dangerous clots by keeping the blood flowing freely. Blood clots, typically in the legs, become a greater danger as you age and mobility decreases, but a few minutes of stretching boosts healthy circulation. Preventative health begins with stretching.

The boost in blood flow elevates energy. As sluggish circulation contributes to fatigue, getting the blood pumping helps you feel more vibrant. Improved circulation delivers benefits from head to toe - including glowing, youthful skin.

4. Stress Reduction

Stretching is helpful for stress relief and relaxation for many seniors. The focused breathing and gentle movements provide a mini meditation session, allowing the mind and body to reset.

Stretching elicits the "relaxation response" by activating the parasympathetic nervous system. This triggers broad physiologic changes: lowering blood pressure, slowing heart rate, and relaxing muscle tension. Therefore, stretching before bed is tremendously calming for seniors with anxiety or insomnia.

Releasing physical tension relieves mental tension. Slow, deep stretches combined with focused breathing give your mind a break from its usual chatter. Anxiety and worries float away as you sink into the sensations of stretching.

Seniors dealing with grief, depression, or loneliness will benefit from stretching's stress-relieving qualities. The movements can get you out of your head and into your body. For a few minutes, inhabit the present rather than dwelling on the past or future. Let go of stress as you stretch.

5. Enhanced Balance and Coordination

Preserving balance and coordination is another crucial benefit of stretching for seniors. Age-related stiffening combined with weakened muscles leads to unsteadiness and increases the risk of falling. However, stretching improves stability in several crucial ways.

First, opening up tight joints through stretching enhances proprioception – your body's sense of its position in space. Accurately sensing the location and movement of your body is integral to maintaining balance. Stretching keeps these neural pathways sharp.

Second, flexible muscles coordinate movements better than tight, stiff muscles. Responsive muscles allow you to react quickly to slips or imbalances, making you less likely to tumble. Stretching strengthens core muscles, which are essential for balance.

Third, stretching reduces tension that constrains optimal alignment. When your body is properly stacked without unnecessary tightness, you gain stability and poise in motion and standing. With stretching, your whole body works together to keep you centered.

6. Mental Clarity

Regular stretching boosts mental clarity in addition to physical agility. Moving and stretching gets the blood flowing to your brain. The increased oxygenation and nutrient delivery energize the mind. Hence, better circulation aids memory and focus.

Many seniors report stretching helps clear "brain fog" and improves concentration. Neurotransmitters like serotonin and dopamine are released during stretching. The happy hormones with reduced stress revitalize mental sharpness. You will retrieve words or focus on tasks much better after stretching.

Furthermore, stretching synchronizes breathing patterns, which optimizes energy and cognitive performance - following the breath in a stretching routine results in greater presence and awareness. With clearer thinking, you can better connect with friends or engage in hobbies.

Safety Considerations for Senior Stretching

Stretching benefits seniors immensely, but establishing safe stretching habits is crucial. Here are key considerations:

1. Consult Your Healthcare Provider

Consulting your physician before embarking on a new exercise routine, including stretching, is advisable. Your doctor can assess your current health status and advise which stretches would be appropriate or inadvisable given your conditions.

Every senior has unique needs, so it's important to identify limitations or precautions you should take. Your doctor can tailor recommendations based on your health history and previous injuries. They can refer you to physical therapists or trainers familiar with safe senior stretching techniques.

2. Warm-Up and Cool Down

Properly warming up and cooling down before and after stretching is crucial for injury prevention. When cold, muscles are stiffer and more vulnerable to tears and strains. Warming up elevates the body's core temperature and increases blood flow to muscles preparing for activity.

Before stretching, devote 5-10 minutes to gentle warm-up movements. Options include walking in place, doing light arm swings across the body, foot, and ankle circles, or marching with high knees. Also, low-impact aerobic activity effectively warms up muscles. The aim is to gradually increase your heart rate, loosen up joints, and prepare your body for stretching.

3. Listen to Your Body

Tuning into your body's signals during stretching is vital for seniors. Pain or discomfort means you must modify the stretch to be gentler on joints and muscles. The safe stretching motto is "mild tension, never pain." Use pain as your warning signal to lighten up or release a stretch completely.

Pay attention to your limits in each stretch. Ease into the stretch until you reach your threshold of mild tension, then hold it there. Avoid forcing mobility your body isn't ready for or trying to push past pain barriers. Over-stretching and muscle damage in seniors take much longer to heal.

4. Balance and Support

Since balance declines with age, utilize external support during standing stretches for stability. All standing stretches should be performed near a wall, sturdy chair, countertop, or other steady surface. Lightly hold onto supports to catch yourself.

If you feel shaky during one-legged standing stretches, keep the unsupported leg hovering above the ground rather than lifting it high. Have a chair or wall nearby for quick support if you're unsteady. Only lower the stretching leg when your standing leg feels solidly rooted.

To maximize stability, stand with your feet hip-width apart, core engaged, knees softly bent, and vision-focused throughout each stretch. Wear supportive, non-slip footwear. Ask a partner or trainer to spot you for added safety until the single-leg standing strengthens.

Chapter 2: The Aging Body

Aging brings changes to the body naturally that must be understood so that you can adapt your lifestyle accordingly. This chapter explores how the aging process affects the body and mobility. Readers learn how stretching can be a valuable tool for seniors to maintain and improve flexibility. Older adults can tailor exercise routines to preserve mobility and comfort by comprehending age-related changes. This knowledge empowers seniors to care for their changing bodies.

Understanding How the Body Changes with Age

The natural aging process affects every system and structure in your body. While some changes are inevitable, understanding what happens physically as you age allows you to make lifestyle adaptations to maximize health. Below are key ways common body areas change with age and how preserving mobility through stretching provides benefits.

1. Loss of Muscle Mass and Strength

One of the most noticeable age-related changes is a steady decline in muscle mass and strength called sarcopenia. This decline occurs due to reduced synthesis of muscle proteins, muscle fibers dying off, and motor neurons degenerating. Loss of fast-twitch muscle fibers is especially pronounced.

Without resistance exercise, muscle mass decreases approximately 3-8% each decade after age 30. This muscle tissue loss leads to weakness, reduced ability to perform functional and daily tasks, impaired balance, slower gait, and increased risk of falls.

However, stretching helps counteract the sarcopenia effects. Although stretching does not build muscle like strength training, regular stretching maintains muscle flexibility and range of motion, allowing you to continue using your muscles more effectively despite strength reductions. Stretching keeps muscles supple for better daily function.

2. Joint Stiffness and Pain

Years of use lead to progressive wear and tear on joints. Cartilage thins and loses elasticity, synovial fluid dries up, and stiffness sets in. Joints lose their smooth gliding motion, leading to pain, swelling, tenderness, and reduced flexibility, and osteoarthritis becomes more common with age.

These joint changes make everyday movements like getting dressed, driving, opening jars, or golfing more difficult. However, stretching improves joint mobility by taking the joints through their full range of motion to maintain cartilage health and lubrication. Also, stretching releases tight muscles, pulling on joints.

For those with arthritis, gently stretching warms up stiff joints while easing associated aches. Simple range of motion exercises reduce arthritis pain and keep joints as mobile as possible despite degenerative changes.

3. Weakening of Bones

Bone density steadily declines with age due to mineral loss and reduced osteoblast formation, making the bones porous, fragile, and susceptible to fractures, known as osteoporosis. Osteoporosis affects over 10 million Americans over 50. Fracturing a bone due to osteoporosis can be life-changing at advanced ages.

While stretching does not reverse osteoporosis, maintaining flexibility and stability through stretching is a vital prevention measure. Stretching strengthens the muscles supporting the skeleton, taking the pressure off the bones. Building balance lowers fall risk and the chances of fractures. Stretching allows individuals with osteoporosis to continue vigorous bone-strengthening activities.

4. Reduced Connective Tissue Elasticity

Tendons and ligaments lose elasticity and shock-absorbing ability over time, leading to tighter muscles, stiff joints, and a reduced range of motion. Thickened, shorter connective tissues are more vulnerable to overuse injuries and tears. However, stretching lengthens these tissues.

For example, stretching the hamstrings after exercise helps maintain length in the leg tendons and muscles. Stretching the shoulder joint capsule and muscles protects ligaments. Regular stretching combats pliability loss in tissues around joints to support a fuller range of motion, protecting against strains and mobility limitations.

5. Postural and Balance Changes

Due to muscle weakness, aging brings postural changes like forward head position, rounded shoulders, and exaggerated back curving. Balance declines with age as joints stiffen and sensory input diminishes. These factors significantly increase seniors' risk of debilitating falls.

However, focused stretching strengthens the muscles, supporting proper upright posture. Stretches that open the chest and strengthen the upper back prevent rounded shoulders. Stability training stretches retrain balance, giving seniors greater confidence in walking and standing and reducing the risk of injury from falls.

6. Cardiovascular Changes

The cardiovascular system also ages. Hardening and losing elasticity in blood vessels lead to hypertension and reduced blood flow. Maximum heart output falls. However, stretching boosts circulation to partially alleviate these cardiovascular changes.

Moving major muscle groups through stretching exercises requires the heart to pump more blood. Stretching increases vascular elasticity and lowers resting blood pressure. The deep breathing coordinated with stretching maximizes oxygen delivery. Therefore, regular stretching maintains essential cardiovascular health as you age.

Common Issues and Limitations in Seniors

The natural physical changes with aging eventually manifest in challenging issues and limitations. Understanding the fundamental problems allows older adults to address these health concerns proactively. Here are the most common age-related issues among seniors:

1. Reduced Range of Motion

One of the most frustrating effects of aging is a progressive loss of range of motion and flexibility. Joints naturally stiffen with age. The tendons, ligaments, and muscles surrounding the joints also become less elastic, restricting mobility.

Limited range of motion primarily impacts the major joints like shoulders, hips, knees, and spine. Simple movements like looking over the shoulder to back up a car, bending to tie shoes, or reaching overhead become more challenging. Restricted mobility makes many routine activities difficult.

Flexibility deficits around the shoulder joint will cause problems. For instance, tightness prevents raising the arms above the head to dress, style hair, or reach for items on a high shelf. Moreover, limited shoulder mobility hinders recreational pursuits like golf, swimming, or racket sports.

Reduced hip and spinal flexibility contributes to balance challenges. Tight hamstrings and hips limit stride length during walking. Rigidity in the spine impacts posture, ability to rotate, and shock absorption. Hence, maintaining a range of motion promotes comfort and function.

2. Stiffness and Discomfort

Joint stiffness and muscle tightness do more than reduce mobility, leading to generalized achiness and discomfort. As joints lose smooth movement, the cartilage wears down, and the bones rub together. Inflammation and swelling stress nerves, causing pain.

Areas most prone to stiffness and arthritis as you age are the knees, hips, hands, and lower back. Just performing simple actions like getting up from a chair, opening a jar, or grasping objects becomes painful. Chronic discomfort and pain sap the motivation to exercise and stay active.

In addition to joint soreness, tight muscles cause discomfort. Shortened tissues strain against bony attachments, leading to muscular pain. Lack of activity allows muscles to further knot up and spasm. Stiffness throughout the body causes a reluctance to move.

Gentle stretching provides relief by lubricating stiff joints and lengthening contracted muscles. Range of motion exercises lessens localized aches while building tolerance for activity. Stretching's benefits motivate seniors to continue being active.

3. Balance Problems

As balance reflexes decline with age, seniors face an increased risk of falling. Falls often lead to serious injury, hospitalization, loss of independence, and reduced quality of life. Therefore, understanding and preventing falls is essential.

Age-related structural and neurological changes impair balance. As joints stiffen, proprioception diminishes, vision worsens, muscles weaken, and maintaining equilibrium during motion or standing becomes difficult. Fast reflexes and coordination also decline.

Weak core muscles and tight hips, hamstrings, and calves lead to balance deficits during everyday activities. Standing on one foot to dress or turning quickly can become impossible without losing stability. Eventually, the fear of falling discourages seniors from normal movement.

However, focused stretching and balance exercises retrain motor control skills while building leg and core strength for poise in motion. Practicing tandem stance and single-leg deadlifts within a safe stretching routine sharpens balance reactions.

4. Loss of Independence

The cumulative impact of decreased flexibility, discomfort, unsteadiness, and reduced mobility is a loss of independence in daily living. Completing personal care tasks or household activities requires increased dependence when basic functional movements become challenging.

Difficulty with steps due to stiff knees and hips forces reliance on railings or walkers. Handling kitchen tasks like opening containers and lifting pots is taxing with arthritic fingers and weak wrists. Equally, dressing, bathing, and grooming pose challenges with limited shoulder mobility.

Mobility loss and falling risks increase dependence on others for community navigation or transportation. Reduced activity tolerance makes hobbies, volunteering, and socializing fatiguing. However, maximizing physical capabilities through stretching sustains independence.

How Stretching Can Address These Issues

The natural effects of aging restricting mobility and comfort do not have to prevent seniors from enjoying active, fulfilling lives. A strategic stretching program can counteract many age-related physical limitations. Regularly performing targeted flexibility exercises preserves range of motion, eases stiffness, improves balance, strengthens muscles, and reduces injury risk.

Here is how consistent stretching successfully combats common issues that develop as you get older:

1. Preserving and Improving Flexibility

One primary benefit of stretching is maintaining and regaining a joint range of motion that naturally diminishes with age. Stretching elongates stiff connective tissues and lubricates joints to preserve healthy mobility.

For example, chest stretches to lengthen tight pectoral muscles allow greater shoulder joint movement for tasks like brushing your hair. Hip flexor stretches to maintain lifting your leg and climbing stairs. Hamstring stretches preserve range so you can bend smoothly.

A full-body stretching routine loosens restricted joints from head to toe. Targeting areas of pronounced stiffness preserves your ability to function independently. Be patient, and you will gradually progress in flexibility over time.

2. Alleviating Muscle and Joint Discomfort

The gentle stretching movements deliver natural pain relief by increasing blood flow to nurture muscles and joints. Improved circulation provides fresh oxygen and nutrients to distressed areas. Stretching further helps realign joints into proper positions to release pressure and discomfort.

Gentle neck stretches alleviate stiffness that causes headaches. Lower back stretches relax muscles that get knotted and pinch nerves. Knee and hip stretches ease arthritis discomfort by lubricating joints and lengthening surrounding tissues. Consistent stretching provides drug-free pain management.

3. Enhancing Balance and Posture

Poor balance and posture result from instability in the musculoskeletal system. Weak muscles cannot properly align and support the body against gravity. Stretching strengthens muscles while opening up proper joint positioning to improve poise.

Moves like single-leg balances work the hip stabilizers. Upper back stretches strengthen the muscles combating forward head positioning. Stretching hip flexors and hamstrings allow the pelvis to tilt into a stable position. The cumulative effect is better balance control and upright, agile posture.

4. Strengthening Muscles

In addition to enhancing flexibility, certain stretching techniques also strengthen the muscles. This helps combat sarcopenia and gives seniors greater stamina for daily activities.

For example, yoga poses, like Warrior I, gently strengthen the quadriceps and glutes in a stretched position. The resistance of bands during standing leg kicks builds lower body strength while improving hip mobility. Tai chi movements strengthen core muscles as you shift your weight through stances. Ultimately, stretching builds supportive muscles.

5. Reducing the Risk of Injury

By improving joint mobility, muscle suppleness, balance control, and postural alignment, stretching significantly reduces seniors' risk of activity-limiting injuries.

Regular stretching protects against strains and sprains by allowing muscles and tendons to move freely through a full range before encountering resistance. Strength developed through stretching makes seniors less prone to falls and fractures. Maintaining flexibility enables continued participation in bone-strengthening exercises.

Chapter 3: Warm-Up and Cooling Down

Properly warming up and cooling down before and after stretching is vital to avoid injury. This chapter shares effective warm-up and cool-down techniques tailored to seniors' needs. You will learn how to prepare for stretching safely and finish your routine. Following proper steps will get you the most flexibility and strength benefits from stretching while protecting your body.

The Significance of Warming Up and Cooling Down

Getting into the habit of warming up before stretching and cooling down afterward is as important as the stretches themselves. Dedicate 5-10 minutes to warm your muscles and raise your heart rate before diving into flexibility exercises.

Similarly, take 5-10 minutes to gradually bring your heart rate down and loosen muscles again after finishing your routine.

Warm-ups and cool-downs are not merely formalities. They are crucial physiological and psychological functions. Let's explore the critical benefits these practices provide older adults to ensure safe, effective stretching.

Warming Up (Pre-Stretching):

Starting your stretching session with a warm-up yields several fundamental benefits that prime your body for mobility exercises and injury prevention. Here are the main purposes for a pre-stretching warm-up:

1. Increased Blood Flow

One core aim of warming up is increasing blood circulation to your resting muscles. Higher blood flow elevates muscle temperature and delivers more oxygen and nutrients. This prepares the muscles for exertion, making them less prone to strain or tear when stretched.

The gentle movements of a warm-up get your blood pumping and enhance vascular flow. Dynamic activities like marching, mini-squats, arm swings, and torso twists accelerate circulation gradually. The increased blood flow also nourishes joint tissues. Warm-ups prime your physiology for action.

2. Enhanced Joint Lubrication

Increased movement and blood supply generated from warming up stimulate the production of synovial fluid. This natural lubricant inside the joints reduces friction and provides smooth joint mobility.

Lubricated joints move more easily through their full range of motion without pain or stiffness. The hips, knees, shoulders, and spine will particularly benefit. Warming up releases tightness by coating joint tissues for better shock absorption.

3. Mental Preparation

Warm-ups allow you to switch gears and be focused mentally. The 3-10 minutes dedicated to gradually raising your heart rate provides the perfect opportunity to set your intention. Warm-ups signal the transition from a sedentary state to activity.

Use the time to relax your muscles consciously, focus on your breath, and center your mind on the present moment. Tune into how your body feels and define your goals, such as a targeted area needing extra flexibility work. Ease into your stretching mindset.

Cooling Down (Post-Stretching):

Like warming up beforehand, cooling down afterward completes your stretching routine effectively. Here are the main benefits of cooling down:

1. Gradual Transition

Cooling down enables a gradual decline in heart rate and blood flow following exertion. It prevents dizziness, lightheadedness, or fainting resulting from sudden heart rate and blood pressure drops after exercise.

Gentle movements like slow walking or gentle joint rotations coupled with deep breathing return your physique to homeostasis safely. The heart rate lowers step-by-step rather than abruptly halting activity. Give your body 5-10 minutes to transition to rest.

2. Muscle Relaxation

Incorporating light static or dynamic stretches during your cool down alleviates muscle tightness built up during your routine. Stretches for the front body, like chest and hip flexors, feel especially good after backward bending.

This post-workout flexibility work helps muscles that shorten and contract during exercise regain normal length and tension. Stretching while muscles are still warm prevents next-day soreness and stiffness. For instance, yoga-style deep breathing enhances the relaxation response.

3. Improved Flexibility

Coordinated stretching as part of your cool down enhances the flexibility gains during your main workout. Muscles that are activated are primed to open further with light-assisted and static stretching.

For example, letting gravity deepen a forward fold stretch after doing standing hamstring stretches, maximizes benefits. Adding stretches at the end of your session maximizes results.

Effective Warm-Up Techniques for Seniors

Getting your blood flowing and muscles warm before stretching is crucial to exercising comfortably and avoiding injury. But with age, you must be more gradual and gentle in warming up than your younger years.

The good news is that 5-10 minutes of simple movements prepare your body for safe, effective stretching. Incorporate these senior-friendly warm-up techniques into your pre-stretching routine to get the most from your workouts.

1. Marching in Place

One of the simplest and most effective warm-ups for seniors is marching in place. This mild aerobic activity gently elevates your heart rate, pumping blood through your resting muscles.

Stand with your feet hip-width apart. Engage your core by drawing your naval in toward your spine. Raise one knee to your chest, swinging the opposite arm forward simultaneously. Alternate lifting your legs and swinging your arms like marching.

Start with a slow, easy tempo. Focus on standing tall, engaging your abs, aligning your knees over your ankles, and breathing deeply. Gradually pick up the pace until you feel your heart rate mildly elevated. Lower knee lifts put less strain on your joints.

You can march in place for 1-3 minutes. Breathe deeply through your nose and drive those knees up and arms back. Marching preps your muscles for action and loosens stiff hips and knees. Make marching the first step of your warm-up.

2. Arm Circles

Now, wake up those upper body muscles. Arm circles open up the shoulders while getting blood flow to your arms and upper back.

Stand comfortably with your feet under your hips, engage your core, relax your shoulders, and point your thumbs forward. Initiate small, gentle circles with your arms, gradually increasing the size. Lead with your thumbs to roll your shoulders back and open up the chest.

Next, turn your thumbs to face backward and circle as though you are touching your back pocket. Bring your shoulder blades together as you lead with your knuckles. This counterbalances the effects of the first direction and works the shoulder joints in all planes of motion.

Start with small circles and go slowly. Focus on control and proper form rather than size. Shoulder injuries are common as you age, so be cautious. Arm circles are excellent pre-workout mobility preparers.

3. Ankle Rolls

It's easy to overlook your feet and ankles during warm-ups, but these joints are crucial shock absorbers during movement. Rolling your ankles increases mobility for safe stepping, walking, and balancing.

Sit tall on a chair or stand, holding on for balance. Rotate your foot clockwise 10 times, moving through the full range of ankle motion. Switch directions and roll counter-clockwise 10 times. Your ankles may feel stiff at first, but keep moving: it reduces the risk of strains down the line.

You can also do ankle rolls while standing on one leg for an added balance challenge. Lightly hold a chair or wall for support. Slowly trace circles with your ankle to wake up those stabilizing muscles. Healthy ankles distribute impact and propel motion.

4. Neck and Shoulder Rolls

Next, address upper body tension with neck and shoulder rolls. Muscles in the neck and shoulders easily tense up, causing stiffness, headaches, and poor posture. Rolling them out prepares for pain-free stretching.

Begin by dropping your chin to your chest. Slowly roll your head to the right across your shoulders toward your armpit. Complete the circle by tipping your head back, then to the left shoulder. Repeat this circle 5 times in one direction, then switch.

For shoulders, raise them toward your ears, then circle them backward and down in 5 rotations. Reverse the roll, pulling shoulders forward, then up. Move slowly and steadily with control. Stop if you feel dizzy. Upper body rolls reduce accumulated tension and strain.

5. Breathing Exercises

No warm-up is complete without belly breathing exercises to connect the mind and body. Deep breathing triggers relaxation, oxygenates your blood, and focuses on intention.

Stand or sit tall and place one hand on your belly. Inhale slowly and deeply through your nose, feeling your belly press into your hand. Exhale slowly out the mouth. Continue this pattern for 1 minute. Close your eyes and focus on your inhalation and exhalation.

Try chanting "Ha" on the exhale to deepen the release. Allow distracting thoughts to float away each time you exhale. Calm, steady breathing preps you for the mental focus to stretch effectively.

Effective Cooling Down Techniques for Seniors

Like warming up beforehand, cooling down properly after stretching is vital. A 5-10 minute cool down transition brings your heart rate down and realigns tissues gently after working them. Don't skip this crucial phase.

Below are highly effective cool-down techniques seniors should integrate. Learn how static stretching, deep breathing, walking, and hydration after workouts ensure you receive full benefits from flexibility training.

1. Static Stretches

Incorporating static stretching as part of your cool-down enhances flexibility results. After taking your muscles through dynamic movements, static holds continue opening joints and lengthening muscles.

Following your main workout, repeat challenging stretches from your routine and hold them statically for 15-30 seconds. For example, if hip flexor stretches are tight, repeat this movement and focus on relaxing into a deeper hold. Or sustain a hamstring stretch after completing dynamic forward folds.

This technique allows muscles to release, relax, and gain length after being stretched dynamically. Pay attention to your breathing, relax rather than force the stretch, and sink deeper into the pose. Your flexibility will improve over time.

Focus on opening particularly tight areas. But listen to your body and back off stretches causing discomfort. While your body is still warm, maximize mobility gains from your session with brief static stretches.

2. Deep Breathing

Let's not forget to integrate deep breathing as part of your cool-down sequence. This grounds your mind, relaxes the nervous system, and directs awareness inward. Make breathing the bridge transitioning from physical exertion to stillness.

Find a comfortable seated position. Close your eyes and place one hand on your belly. Inhale slowly and deeply through your nose into your abdomen, feeling it expand with air. Exhale slowly out through pursed lips.

Repeat this pattern for 2-5 minutes as your heart rate decreases. Visualize tension releasing from your muscles as you exhale. Optional chanting of a sound like "Om" deepens the relaxation response. Make deep breathing the norm during your cool down.

3. Gentle Walking

Low-intensity walking after your stretching routine helps safely bring down your heart rate and blood pressure, preventing dangerous spikes and drops that may occur if you abruptly stop moving.

Take a 5-minute stroll around your home or neighborhood to transition your circulation gently back to resting levels. Maintain deep breathing as you walk to maximize calming benefits. Keep your pace leisurely.

Outdoor walking gives you the added benefit of sunlight and fresh air. But indoors also works. Perhaps do laps around rooms or up and down stairs. Gentle walking concludes your workout safely.

4. Hydration

Always replace fluids after your workout by drinking water or an electrolyte sports drink. Stretching may not seem as intensely hydration-draining as other exercises. However, you still lose water through sweat and respiration.

Adequate hydration allows your heart to pump freshly oxygenated blood through your tissues to aid recovery. It replaces electrolytes like sodium and potassium lost in sweat. Drink at least 8 oz. of water after stretching.

Proper hydration reduces next-day muscle soreness and joint stiffness. Controlling thirst ensures you don't overdo activities and become dehydrated. Make rehydrating part of your post-stretching ritual.

Properly warming up and cooling down before and after stretching is crucial. These practices help seniors maximize flexibility gains from exercises while preventing injury. Stretching becomes more beneficial and enjoyable with wise preparation.

Chapter 4: Upper Body Stretches

This chapter focuses on senior-friendly upper body stretches. Flexibility in your neck, shoulders, arms, and chest is essential for everyday activities like reaching, lifting, and hugging. Limited mobility makes these actions challenging. The stretches in this chapter target upper body areas to improve seniors' range of motion and comfort. Follow along carefully. If neck or back stretches cause dizziness, only continue them while seated. With gentle, regular stretching, seniors can regain ease of movement in their upper body for daily life and enjoyment.

Neck, Shoulder, and Upper Back Stretches

1. Neck Stretch:

The neck is prone to tension and limited mobility as you age. Stretching keeps this area limber for pain-free movement. Here's how to do the neck stretch:

1. Start by sitting or standing tall with a good upright posture. Engage your core muscles and keep your chin level, eyes looking ahead.

2. Gently lower your right ear toward your right shoulder. Take your time, no sudden movements. Support your head with your hand if necessary.

3. Feel a mild stretch on the right side of your neck. You're not trying to tear your head off. Hold and breathe for 15-30 seconds.

4. Bring your head back to the center, then repeat to the left side. Again, take it slow and gentle.

5. Go back and forth, stretching the neck carefully side to side about 2-3 reps each. This stretch loosens up the neck over time.

2. Shoulder Rolls:

Next, open up those tight shoulders. Rolling and stretching keep shoulders mobile and improve posture. Here's how to do shoulder rolls:

1. Start by sitting or standing tall with arms relaxed by your sides. No hunching forward.

2. Initiate shoulder rolls by raising them toward your ears. Control the motion as you roll them backward and down.

3. Once they complete a circle, roll back, reverse, and roll forward, up toward your ears, then down.

4. Repeat for 10-15 rolls backward and 10-15 forward. Ensure full mobility in all directions.

5. You can raise one arm straight, bend the elbow, and stretch it across your chest. Use the other hand to deepen the stretch gently.

6. Hold each shoulder stretch for 15-30 seconds. Remember to breathe. Do 2-3 reps on each side to open the fronts of the shoulders.

3. Upper Back Stretch:

Also, you need to open the tight upper back. Poor posture compresses this area - stretching decompresses. Here's how to do upper back stretch:

1. Sit or stand tall with engaged core muscles. Bring arms straight in front of you.

2. Interlace your fingers together with palms facing outward. Inhale and lengthen arms forward.

3. Exhale and round your upper back, feeling a stretch across your shoulders. Avoid crunching your lower back.

4. Hold the stretch for 15-30 seconds, inhale, and return arms forward to release.

5. Repeat this upper back stretch 2-3 times. Your upper back will feel great after hunching over all day.

Arm and Wrist Stretches

4. Arm Raises:

Arm raises are a simple yet effective exercise to improve arm strength and mobility. As you age, it becomes increasingly important to maintain strength in your arms and shoulders to perform daily tasks and retain independence. Arm raises target the shoulders' deltoid muscles and the upper arms' biceps and triceps muscles.

To perform arm raises:

1. Stand or sit tall with good posture, keeping your core engaged. Make sure your feet are hip-width apart if standing.

2. Let your arms relax at your sides. Raise one arm straight in front of you up to shoulder height. Keep the arm straight throughout the movement.

3. Slowly lower the arm back to the starting position. Repeat with the other arm.

4. Lift the arm using control - avoid swinging or jerking motions. Keep breathing throughout the exercise.

5. Complete 5-10 controlled raises with each arm. Go at your own pace.

6. Focus on using the shoulder muscles to lift the arm up and down in a smooth, controlled motion. Keep the elbow straight and the wrist neutral.

7. Start with a light or no weight. You can hold a small hand weight or canned good once you build strength.

8. Arm raises strengthen the shoulder muscles, assisting in daily tasks like brushing hair, reaching up to shelves, carrying bags, and dressing.

9. Regular arm raises help keep shoulders mobile and flexible to support a pain-free range of motion. They provide cardio benefits by getting the blood pumping.

10. Take care not to overdo it. Listen to your body. Start slowly and build up as you gain strength. Proper form is vital.

11. Make sure to work the back of the shoulders with rows or reverse flys to balance the muscles worked.

Arm raises are a simple addition to an exercise routine, providing significant benefits. Focus on controlled, proper form, and be patient as you build shoulder strength. Consistency is key. Aim for arm raises 2-3 times a week to maintain mobility.

5. Wrist Flexor Stretch:

Stretching the muscles and joints in the wrists and forearms to relieve tension, improve flexibility, and prevent injury is important. The wrist flexor stretch targets the muscles on the underside of the forearm that bend the wrist downward. Regularly performing this stretch helps maintain wrist mobility.

To do the wrist flexor stretch:

1. Stand or sit tall with a good upright posture. Extend one arm straight in front of you with the palm facing down toward the floor.

2. With your other hand, gently grasp the extended hand and fingers. Slowly bend the wrist down gently until you feel a mild stretch on the underside of the forearm.

3. Hold the stretch for 15-30 seconds. Breathe deeply and avoid overstretching to the point of pain. A mild tension is ideal.

4. Release the stretch and shake out the wrist. Repeat 2-3 times on each wrist. Switch arms and stretch the other wrist.

5. You can use a towel or strap around the fingers of the extended hand to provide a gentle downward pull if needed.

6. Stretch both wrists evenly. Do not hyperextend the wrist joint.

7. Aim to do this stretch 2-3 times a week to maintain flexibility in the wrist flexor muscles.

8. If you spend much time with your wrists bent, as in computer work, stretching is extra important to counter tightness.

9. Listen to your body and back off if you feel sharp pain. Pain is a warning sign to stop. Mild tension is normal and desired.

10. Proper wrist flexor stretching can help relieve tension from repetitive gripping motions and relieve associated wrist soreness or pain.

11. Work on wrist and forearm stretches equally to maintain flexibility on all sides.

Stretching the wrist flexors is simple and substantially benefits wrist comfort and function. Take time to gently target these muscles 2-3 times a week. Proper stretching promotes wrist health and flexibility for everyday tasks.

6. Wrist Extensor Stretch:

Like stretching the wrist flexors, stretching the extensor muscles on the top of the forearm that extend the wrist is also important. Tight extensors can contribute to wrist stiffness and soreness. This stretch provides relief.

To perform the wrist extensor stretch:

1. Stand or sit upright with good posture. Extend one arm straight in front of you with the palm facing up to the ceiling.

2. With your other hand, gently grasp the extended hand and fingers. Slowly bend the hand downward until you feel a mild stretch along the topside of the forearm.

3. Hold for 15-30 seconds, breathing deeply. Avoid overstretching to the point of pain. Mild tension is ideal.

4. Release the stretch and shake out the wrist. Repeat 2-3 times on each wrist. Switch arms.

5. You can also loop a towel or strap around the extended fingers to provide traction if needed. Avoid pulling too forcefully.

6. Stretch both wrists evenly. Do not hyperextend the joint backward. Keep the stretch gentle.

7. Aim to stretch the wrist extensors 2-3 times a week to maintain flexibility and counter tightness.

8. This stretch counters tightness caused by repetitive wrist extension, such as in backhand motions in sports like tennis.

9. Listen to your body and back off if you feel sharp pain. Mild tension is normal and desired.

Combine stretching the wrist extensors and flexors to maintain balance and comfort. Proper stretching can help prevent and relieve wrist soreness related to overuse and repetitive motions.

Chest and Abdominal Stretches

7. Chest Opener:

The chest opener is an excellent stretch to relieve chest and front shoulder tightness. Poor posture and inactivity can cause the chest muscles to tighten, resulting in rounded shoulders and poor posture. Regularly stretching the chest helps counteract these effects.

To perform the chest opener stretch:

1. Stand or sit tall with an upright posture. Engage your core. Keep your chin tucked and shoulders down.

2. Reach both arms straight behind you, crossing one hand over the other at the wrists or clasping hands together, if able.

3. Gently squeeze your shoulder blades together while lifting your chest. Avoid arching your lower back.

4. You should feel a mild stretch across your chest and front shoulders. Hold for 15-30 seconds, breathing deeply.

5. Release the stretch and relax the arms. Repeat 2-3 times.

6. Go slowly and avoid overarching the back. The stretch should feel mild - not painful.

7. Focus on keeping the shoulders down and the chest lifted throughout. Do not strain.

8. Start with a smaller range of motion and work up to bigger stretches as your flexibility increases.

9. Be patient and consistent. Do this stretch 2-3 times a week to maintain chest mobility.

10. Pair chest opening with upper back stretches like rows or reverse flys.

11. If needed, you can use a towel or strap around the hands behind the back to assist this stretch.

Proper chest stretching can help relieve tightness, improve posture, and allow fuller breaths. A more open, flexible chest can reduce pressure and discomfort.

8. Abdominal Stretch:

The seated back arch is a simple stretch providing mobility through the upper back, chest, and abdomen.

To perform this stretch:

1. Sit tall on a sturdy, armless chair with your feet flat on the floor. Maintain a good upright posture. Engage your core.

2. Hold onto the sides of the chair for support and stability. Keep your shoulders back.

3. Inhale and gently arch your back, leaning slightly backward. Avoid crunching or overarching the lower back.

4. You should feel a mild stretch across your chest and front of your abdomen. Breathe deeply.

5. Hold this arched-back position for 15-30 seconds. Find a mild tension without overdoing it.

6. Exhale and slowly release the stretch by returning to an upright seated posture. Relax your back.

7. Repeat this back-arching sequence 2-3 times. Move carefully and with control.

8. Start with small back arches and work up to bigger stretches as your flexibility allows. Listen to your body.

9. Holding the chair provides stability to support the stretch safely. Keep your core engaged.

10. Avoid painful overarching. The stretch should feel mild to moderately tense but not painful.

11. Be patient and do this stretch consistently 2-3 times a week for flexibility gains.

12. This stretch helps open the chest and front of the torso, improving posture and balance.

13. Counteracting a hunched posture can relieve upper back tightness and pressure.

Incorporating these upper body stretches into your daily routine will keep your neck, shoulders, arms, and chest flexible as you continue your stretching journey. Regularly performing exercises for these areas enhances your range of motion and reduces discomfort from tightness. Improved mobility makes everyday activities more manageable and enjoyable, contributing to your overall well-being.

Chapter 5: Lower Body Stretches

Flexibility and strength in the lower body are vital to maintain mobility and independence as you age. Your legs enable you to perform essential daily activities, from walking to climbing stairs. This chapter explores stretches targeting the legs, ankles, calves, hips, and lower back. Regularly performing these exercises improves the range of motion and keeps the lower body limber to support an active lifestyle.

Leg and Thigh Stretches

Keeping the legs flexible and limber is essential for maintaining mobility and stability as you age. The large muscle groups in the thighs and legs enable you to perform vital daily activities from walking to bending down. Without adequate flexibility in these muscles, movements can become difficult, strained, and uncomfortable. The following leg stretches are simple exercises that can be performed safely, providing substantial benefits for improving and maintaining flexibility.

1. **Quadriceps Stretch:**

The quadriceps are the large muscle group on the front of the thighs crucial for extending the knees in everyday functions, like walking, climbing stairs, and transitioning from sitting to standing. Knee mobility and function are negatively impacted when the quadriceps muscles become tight or stiff from lack of use or normal aging. Regularly performing quadriceps stretches helps maintain flexibility and range of motion in these important muscles.

To perform a safe and effective quadriceps stretch:

1. Stand behind a steady chair or wall for support and stability and engage your core muscles.

2. Lift one foot behind you and gently grasp the ankle with your hand. Keep both knees pointing forward and close together.

3. Gently pull the heel toward your buttocks, keeping the thighs aligned and facing forward.

4. You should feel a mild to moderate stretch in the front of the thigh. Remember to breathe deeply.

5. Hold the stretching position for 15-30 seconds, release, and repeat on the other leg.

6. Complete 2-3 controlled stretches on each leg. Move slowly and focus on good form.

7. Be careful not to arch or twist your back during the move. Keep the stretch focused on the quadriceps muscles.

Start with gentle stretches and progress with more intensity as the quads' flexibility improves. Listen to your body.

Stretching the quadriceps helps maintain the mobility of the knees for daily activities, like walking, climbing stairs, and sitting-standing transitions.

Tightness in the quadriceps can contribute to knee discomfort and muscular imbalance between the legs. Consistently stretch them to keep the quads flexible and limber.

2. Hamstring Stretch:

The hamstrings refer to the muscle group located on the back of the thighs that is essential in knee flexion and hip extension. When the hamstrings become overly tight or stiff, mobility in the legs is hindered, and low back tightness is also possible. Regularly stretching the hamstrings is key for maintaining optimal flexibility and function.

To perform an effective hamstring stretch:

1. Sit on a chair with one foot planted firmly on the ground in front of you. Extend the other leg out straight with the heel resting on the floor.

2. Keeping the extended leg straight, lean forward slowly from the hips until you feel a mild to moderate stretch sensation down the back of the thigh. Avoid rounding the lower back.

3. Hold the stretched position for 15-30 seconds, breathing deeply, release, and repeat 2-3 times on each leg.

4. Maintain a good upright posture while doing the move. Keep the stretch focused on the hamstring muscles.

5. You can use a towel looped around the foot for a deeper stretch if needed. Gently pull back to increase tension.

Gradually build the intensity of your stretches as the hamstring flexibility improves. Avoid overstretching.

Stretching improves flexibility in the hamstrings for movements like bending and helps maintain knee function, taking the pressure off the lower back muscles.

3. Inner Thigh Stretch:

The inner thigh adductor muscles enable you to draw your legs inward toward the body's midline. The hips' mobility can be restricted when these muscles tighten with age. Regularly stretching the inner thighs helps open the hips for easy movement.

To safely perform an inner thigh stretch:

1. Sit on a sturdy chair with your back straight and feet flat on the floor.

2. Keep your upper body upright with the core muscles engaged. Exhale and relax the body.

3. Slowly open your legs wider, gently pressing your knees outward to the sides.

4. You should feel a mild to moderate stretch sensation along the inner thighs toward the groin area. Avoid overstretching.

5. Hold the stretched position for 15-30 seconds, breathing deeply. Bring your legs back together and relax.

6. Repeat the sequence 2-3 times and listen to your body.

Avoid pain or pinching sensations. The stretch should produce only mild to moderate tension.

Be patient and continue stretching consistently 2-3 times a week for steady flexibility gains.

This inner thigh stretch promotes hip mobility for everyday movements like getting in and out of a car.

Flexible inner thighs support leg and hip comfort when walking, bending, or fully extending the legs.

Ankle and Calf Stretches

Targeting the ankles and calves with stretches keeps these key areas mobile as you age. Simple exercises like ankle circles and calf stretches, promote flexibility below the knee to aid in walking, balance, getting up from chairs, and going up and down stairs.

4. Ankle Circles:

Maintaining ankle flexibility and mobility as you age is imperative. The ankle joints enable you to walk, climb stairs, and stand from a seated position. Ankle circles are a simple exercise to lubricate the ankles and enhance mobility.

To do ankle circles:

1. Sit in a chair with your feet flat on the floor. Maintain good posture.

2. Lift one foot slightly off the ground, keeping the knee bent. Slowly rotate your ankle clockwise in a circular motion.

3. Complete 10-15 controlled circles moving through your full range of motion, keeping the movements smooth.

4. Reverse the direction and complete 10-15 counterclockwise circles with the same ankle.

5. Switch and repeat the ankle circles with the other ankle, rotating in both directions.

Ankle circles help lubricate the joint space and warm up the ankle for increased mobility. This exercise promotes ankle flexibility for walking, standing up, and balance.

Stiff ankles can lead to strained movements and an increased risk of falls. Stretch them regularly. Start with a few circles and gradually increase the reps as the ankle flexibility improves.

5. Calf Stretch:

Tight, stiff calf muscles can restrict ankle mobility, making walking painful. Regularly stretching the calves helps maintain a normal range of motion.

To stretch the calves:

1. Stand facing a wall for support. Place one foot forward and one foot back.

2. Keep the back leg straight with the heel on the floor and the front leg bent.

3. Lean forward, pressing the back heel into the floor until you feel a stretch in the calf.

4. Hold for 15-30 seconds, breathing deeply. Repeat 2-3 times on each side.

5. The back knee can be slightly bent, but avoid bending so that the back heel lifts.

6. Keep your torso upright to avoid rounding the lower back. Focus on the stretch below the knee.

7. If needed, use a towel under the ball of the foot for a deeper stretch. Gently pull back.

Consistently stretch the calf muscles to maintain ankle mobility for walking and other activities. Flexible calves help prevent foot cramps and aid in balance and stability.

Hip and Lower Back Stretches

Keeping the hip and lower back areas limber and flexible is key for maintaining mobility as you age. Tightness and stiffness in the hip muscles and lower back can make everyday movements like bending, getting dressed, picking up objects from the floor, or reaching overhead challenging and uncomfortable. Regularly doing simple stretches focused on the hips and lower back helps improve the range of motion and reduces strain in these critical areas.

6. Hip Flexor Stretch:

The hip flexor muscles pull the knee upward and enable lifting your legs. When these muscles become overly tight or stiff, mobility in the hips is restricted, and the range of motion for leg movements is reduced. Consistently stretching the hip flexors helps open the hips for easier motion.

To perform an effective hip flexor stretch:

1. Stand tall with your feet about hip-width apart for stability. Engage your core muscles.

2. Step one leg back with the knee bent at 90 degrees. Be careful not to lean forward at the hips.

3. Keeping the torso upright, gently tilt your pelvis forward. You will feel a mild to moderate stretch sensation in the front of the hip area.

4. Hold this stretched position for 15-30 seconds, breathing deeply. Slowly return to the starting position and repeat 2-3 times on each leg.

5. Focus on maintaining a good upright posture throughout the stretching movement. Avoid arching or rounding the spine.

Start with small, gentle stretches and gradually increase the intensity as your hip flexibility improves. Listen to your body.

Stretching the hip flexors improves mobility for movements like high stepping, striding out, and bending comfortably.

It allows a greater range of motion in the hips and reduces strain on the lower back muscles.

7. Lower Back Stretch:

Tightness and stiffness commonly develop in the lower back muscles as you age. Gently stretching the lower back area can relieve muscle tension and improve the overall range of motion.

To safely perform a lower back stretch:

1. Sit toward the front of a sturdy chair with feet together flat on the floor. Maintain a good upright posture.

2. Bend one knee and cross the ankle over the opposite knee.

3. Gently lean forward from the hips and press down on the crossed knee to create a mild to moderate stretch in the lower back.

4. Hold the stretch for 15-30 seconds, breathing deeply, release, and repeat 2-3 times on each side.

5. Start with gentle stretches and increase the intensity as your lower back flexibility improves.

6. Be careful not to round the spine during the move. Keep the neck and back straight.

7. After stretching, bring both feet together and do gentle spinal twists for additional relief.

Incorporating lower body stretches for the legs, hips, back, ankles, and calves into your daily routine enhances flexibility in these fundamental areas as you continue your senior stretching journey. Regularly performing exercises targeting the lower body improves mobility, reduces discomfort, and enables performing daily activities with greater comfortability and independence for better overall well-being.

Chapter 6: Balance and Stability Exercises

Balance and stability are critical for seniors to maintain independence and avoid falls. Stretching for seniors encompasses flexibility exercises and movements that enhance balance. This chapter explores the importance of balance and introduces exercises specifically for improving steadiness on the feet by training the muscles that contribute to equilibrium and stability.

Importance of Balance for Seniors

As you age, balance becomes increasingly vital for staying steady on your feet, preventing falls, and maintaining independence in daily life. Balance is maintaining proper upright posture and equilibrium when performing various movements, such as walking, bending, standing up, reaching overhead, or transitioning between positions. For seniors specifically, good balance serves several crucial functions:

1. **Fall Prevention**

Falls are a significant concern among senior citizens and can lead to serious injuries, such as hip fractures, head trauma, broken bones, and other conditions requiring hospitalization. Loss of balance is a major contributing factor to falling. A strong balance minimizes the risk of a dangerous tumble. Proper stability when standing or walking ensures seniors have the requisite control to avoid losing their footing unexpectedly.

Enhancing balance through specific exercises strengthens the muscles in the core, hips, legs, and ankles, contributing to steadiness on the feet, which is fundamental for fall prevention. Balance relies on multiple harmonious physical systems, including the brain, vision, inner ear, muscles, joints, and proprioception. If one or more of these systems degrade, the balance declines.

Common factors that erode balance in older adults include:

- Age-related muscle weakness in the lower body.

- Neurological conditions like Parkinson's disease.

- Arthritis and joint stiffness.

- Diminished vision or vestibular problems in the inner ear.

- Side effects of certain medications.

- Poor posture

- Lack of balance training.

Improving balance through exercise counteracts these issues and bolsters stability. Advanced age diminishes balance through natural physiological decline. However, targeted training helps maintain equilibrium even into the senior years. Proper balance enables seniors to catch themselves more readily if they start to fall. It builds leg strength to arrest a fall before it happens. Solid balance is the first line of defense for fall prevention for the elderly.

2. Independence

Another essential benefit of good balance for seniors is maintaining independence in everyday activities. Balance allows older adults to confidently and safely perform functions like getting dressed, bathing, using the stairs, reaching down to pick up objects, walking the dog, or doing household chores without fear of falling or needing assistance. A steady gait allows seniors to live autonomously and unassisted.

Maintaining the ability to walk safely prevents the need for walkers, canes, or wheelchairs, enabling seniors to get around their homes and communities independently. This freedom of movement is essential for physical health and mental well-being. Balance training also aids in recovery after illness, surgery, or hospitalization to get seniors back on their feet. Stability, strength, and equilibrium are essential for preserving independence as you age.

3. Quality of Life

Additionally, balance directly impacts the overall quality of life for seniors. Being steady on your feet provides the confidence and ability to be active and engaged in social functions, hobbies, volunteer work, and leisure pursuits that bring joy. Seniors with poor balance often limit their activities and interactions to avoid falling, leading to isolation, depression, and loss of purpose.

Good equilibrium allows older adults to fully participate in the things they love without restriction, like dancing, traveling, exercising, playing with grandchildren, or attending community events. Balance reduces the risk of fractures and musculoskeletal injuries that could hamper mobility. Therefore, maintaining balance through the senior years preserves life satisfaction, well-being, and mental health.

Balance Exercises to Complement Stretching

Incorporating balance and stability exercises into your stretching routine can significantly improve your equilibrium and steadiness on your feet. Balance relies on multiple physical systems working in harmony, including vision, inner ear, muscles, joints, and proprioception. If one or more of these systems is compromised, the balance declines. Dedicated balance training counteracts many age-related changes to these systems that can throw off equilibrium. Here are highly effective balance exercises for seniors:

1. **Single-Leg Stance**

The single-leg stance is one of the simplest yet most effective balance drills. It involves standing on one leg, forcing the ankles, calves, hips, and core muscles to activate to avoid toppling over.

To do the single-leg stance:

1. Lean on a wall or chair if you need support. Engage your core.

2. Lift one foot slightly off the ground, bending the knee for stability, and balancing on the other leg.

3. Maintain the position without wavering or needing external support. Hold for 10-15 seconds.

4. Slowly lower the raised foot and switch to balancing on the other leg. Repeat.

5. Start with short intervals and gradually increase the single-leg standing time as you get steadier.

6. Always keep external support handy until you build confidence in your balance.

This exercise strengthens the muscles that maintain equilibrium and stability. Single-leg standing improves posture, ankle strength, and coordination. Make this move part of your daily routine for significant improvements in balance.

2. Heel-to-Toe Walking

Heel-to-toe walking involves taking small steps, precisely placing the heel of one foot directly in front of the other foot's toes, like walking on a tightrope. This challenges your balance and stability.

To do the heel-to-toe walk:

1. Begin in a standing position with a good upright posture. Engage your core muscles.

2. Take an initial small step, putting one foot directly in front of the other by lining up the heel and toes.

3. Continue taking tiny, careful steps, placing the feet heel to toe with each step.

4. Focus on maintaining your balance and a straight line as you walk forward.

5. Take 10-20 heel-to-toe steps forward, then reverse directions and walk backward 10-20 steps.

6. Keep the movements slow and controlled. Stop and regain balance if needed.

7. Use a wall or chair for hand support until you build confidence.

8. Start on level ground before progressing to uneven terrain.

Heel-to-toe walking improves coordination, proprioception, posture, and leg strength, enhancing balance. Make this fun drill part of your routine 2-3 times a week.

3. Flamingo Stand

This unique balance exercise improves uni-pedal (single-leg) balance. Maintaining the flamingo position challenges core stability.

To do the flamingo stand:

1. Stand near a steady wall or chair in case you require hand support. Engage your core.

2. Bend one knee and grasp the ankle with your hand.

3. Gently pull the ankle toward your buttocks while balancing on the other leg.

4. Avoid rounding your spine. Stay tall. Keep the abdominal muscles tight.

5. Maintain the flamingo position for 10-15 seconds before releasing the leg gently.

6. Shake out the standing leg and switch sides, repeating the sequence on the other leg.

7. Use your fingertips on the wall or chair back to aid balance only as needed.

8. Start with brief intervals and increase the single-leg balance as you progress.

The flamingo stand improves lower body strength, proprioception, and stability to enhance overall balance. Make this unique drill a regular part of your training 2-3 times a week.

4. Balancing on One Foot with Arm Movements

This exercise combines balance on one leg with upper body motions to challenge stability in new ways. The arm movements alter your center of gravity, forcing the standing leg to work harder.

To do this exercise:

1. Stand tall on one leg, lifting the other foot off the floor. Have a chair or wall handy for support.

2. Engage your core muscles. Focus on maintaining an upright posture.

3. Extend both arms straight out to the sides, then up overhead while balancing.

4. Hold the top position for a few seconds before lowering your arms and repeating.

5. Complete 10-15 controlled repetitions while keeping the standing leg stable.

6. Switch to the other leg and repeat.

7. Start by using a wall or chair for hand support until you're steady enough to balance independently.

This move improves unilateral balance, torso stability, coordination, and proprioception. Make it part of your routine 2-3 times a week to maintain and build balance.

5. Tai Chi or Yoga for Balance

Consider participating in tai chi or yoga classes explicitly for seniors in addition to your independent balance training. These mind-body practices incorporate controlled, flowing movements that challenge and improve balance, flexibility, and strength in seniors.

Tai chi uses graceful, dance-like poses integrated with focused breathing and meditation. Holding the various stances develops lower body strength, while the transitions between poses enhance equilibrium and stability.

Yoga for seniors blends gentle stretching, core strengthening, and balancing postures into a holistic practice. Partnering breathing with the moves improves mindfulness, circulation, posture, and steadiness.

The social support and guidance of an instructor in tai chi and yoga classes create accountability and progression. However, balance benefits can be achieved by practicing independently at home using videos or online resources dedicated to seniors.

Safety Tips for Balance Exercises

Improving balance is crucial as you age to prevent falls and maintain mobility. Balance exercises effectively enhance stability and coordination. However, performing balance training safely, especially for older adults or those with balance impairments, is vital. Follow these tips to exercise your balance carefully and progressively:

1. Use Support When Necessary:

Balance exercises can be challenging at first. Don't hesitate to use a sturdy chair, countertop, barre, or wall for support when starting a new balance routine. Lightly hold onto the support structure to help you feel steady as you lift one leg or transition between positions. As your balance, strength, and confidence improve, you can reduce your reliance on the support.

Aim to use support minimally, only with the fingertips when needed. If you're gripping firmly or leaning your full weight on the support, it's a sign to keep practicing at that level. The goal is to balance independently, but don't progress too quickly before you're ready. Support is a safety net to prevent falls and injuries.

Choosing supportive structures of the correct height is essential. For example, make sure a chair or bench is at a height where you can lightly rest your hand while standing straight. A barre should be around hip height. Door frames and walls often work well for balance support, but avoid anything unsteady, or that causes you to hunch over.

2. Proper Footwear:

The proper footwear is key for balance training. Wear supportive, comfortable athletic shoes or sneakers with a non-slip sole. Avoid exercise sandals, flats, or shoes with a thick platform or high heel. You want flexible, thin soles with decent tread to allow your feet to sense the floor and grip properly. Make sure the shoes lace snugly and aren't loose around the heel. Properly fitted footwear enhances balance control and stability.

Consider doing balance exercises like tai chi, yoga, or gentle gym routines barefoot. Feeling the floor under your bare feet challenges you to naturally balance while working the tiny stabilizing muscles in the feet. But ensure the exercise surface is completely debris-free, doesn't have trip hazards, and provides traction against slips. Avoid wearing only socks, which can be slippery. Go barefoot or wear athletic shoes.

If you have specific foot problems, like flat feet, bunions, or neuropathy, consult your doctor about therapeutically supportive shoes or inserts to aid balance. Proper footwear optimizes grounding, posture, and alignment when training your equilibrium.

3. Focus on Form:

Pay close attention to your form during balance exercises. Posture and positioning impact your center of gravity, which is critical for balance. Stand or sit tall with an elongated spine, relaxed shoulders, and neck aligned over your torso. Engage your core. Distribute weight evenly between both feet, and don't lock your knees.

When shifting positions, move slowly, smoothly, and controlled. Gradually adjust your stance or the positioning of your arms to stay centered. Don't make sudden, jerky changes. Suspend movements for a moment to regain stability before proceeding if necessary. Moving mindfully with good form minimizes wobbling.

Focus your gaze straightforwardly, not down at your feet. Pick a point ahead of you to spot and keep your eyes anchored there. Also, be mindful not to extend your neck or rounded shoulders, which can throw you off balance. Proper alignment from head to toe gives you a strong support base.

Avoid leaning your torso to the stance side if doing unilateral exercises standing on one leg. Shift your hips over your standing leg rather than bending your spine. Keep your mass center directly over the supporting leg for optimal stability. Practicing balancing evenly on both sides is imperative. Focusing on good form builds proper technique and prevents injury.

4. Be Consistent:

Consistency is critical for improving balance over the long term. Incorporate balance exercises into your routine several days a week for at least 10-15 minutes each session. Regularly training your equilibrium maximizes adaptation.

Vary your exercises to challenge balance from every angle - forward and backward, side-to-side, up and down, static holds, dynamic transitions, on unstable surfaces, while moving, etc. Work on exercises targeting personal balance deficits to improve. Moreover, integrate balance routines as part of your warm-up and cool-down when strength training.

Balance is a skill requiring continual use or lose-it practice. It's common for equilibrium abilities to decline after an illness, vacation, or hiatus from regular training. Be patient and persistent in regaining the balance ground you've lost. Staying consistent with equilibrium activities makes balancing habits natural and ongoing.

Chapter 7: Chair-Based Stretches

For some seniors, mobility limitations or balance concerns may make standing exercises challenging. In these cases, chair-based stretches are a valuable alternative. Seated exercises can improve flexibility, reduce discomfort, and enhance well-being without standing.

Stretches While Sitting

1. Seated Neck Stretch:

1. Sit upright on the front half of a chair with feet flat on the floor.

2. Gently tilt your head to one side, bringing your ear toward the shoulder. Avoid crunching your neck forward.

3. Hold the stretch for 15-30 seconds, breathing deeply.

4. Lift your head back to the center and tilt to the other side.

5. Repeat 2-3 times on each side.

This seated neck stretch relieves tension, increases cervical mobility, and combats forward head posture.

2. Seated Shoulder Rolls:

1. Sit tall with your back straight, feet flat, and hands in your lap.

2. Initiate movement from the shoulders as you roll them up, forward, down, and back in a circular motion.

3. Repeat for 10-15 rolls in each direction.

Rolling shoulders release upper back and rotator cuff tightness.

3. **Seated Arm and Back Stretch:**

    1. Sit upright with feet flat and hands clasped in front.

    2. Inhale while reaching arms overhead.

    3. Exhale while extending your arms forward and rounding your upper back. Feel the chest and abdominal stretch.

    4. Hold for 15-30 seconds, then release with control.

    5. Repeat 2-3 times.

This stretch lengthens the shoulders, chest, and spinal erectors.

4. **Seated Leg Extension:**

    1. Begin by sitting toward the front of a chair with your back straight and feet flat.

2. Extend one leg directly forward, keeping the leg active by flexing the ankle.

3. Hold for 10-15 seconds, breathing deeply and feeling the stretch in the back of your thigh.

4. Lower your leg and switch sides. Repeat 2-3 times with each leg.

Simple seated leg extensions target the hamstrings.

5. **Seated Ankle Circles:**

1. Sit upright with your feet flat and hands on your thighs.

2. Lift one foot slightly off the floor.

3. Make controlled circular motions with the ankle in both directions.

4. Complete 10-15 circles in each direction.

5. Switch feet and repeat on the opposite ankle.

These dynamic circles boost ankle mobility and range of motion.

6. **Seated Torso Twist:**

1. Sit tall with your feet flat and hands grasping the chair's edge.

2. Keeping the hips still, gently rotate your upper body toward one side.

3. Hold the twist for 15-30 seconds, breathing deeply.

4. Return to the center, then twist to the opposite side.

5. Repeat 2-3 times on each side.

Controlled twisting increases spinal flexibility, aids digestion, and relieves tension.

Benefits and Considerations

Chair stretches are merely doing gentle stretching exercises from a seated position in a sturdy, secure chair. Moving major muscle groups and joints through their full range of motion while seated enhances flexibility. It allows older adults to gain the advantages of stretching without struggling with standing or lying on the floor.

Chair stretching routines target common problem areas that tighten and lose mobility with age, including the neck, shoulders, upper and lower back, hips, legs, ankles, and feet. Seated stretches can be done as part of a structured routine or integrated spontaneously throughout the day.

Seniors should choose stretches that address their tight or painful areas. Adapting movements around joint replacements or issues like arthritis may require additional modifications. Working with a physical therapist or fitness professional trained in senior stretching can help identify the best chair exercises for individual needs and abilities.

Benefits of Seated Stretching for Seniors

Performing gentle stretches while seated in a stable chair offers older adults a low-impact way to improve flexibility. Chair stretching increases the range of motion without the strain or fall risks of standing positions.

Here are the main advantages of chair-based stretches for seniors:

1. Accessibility

One of the most significant benefits of chair stretching is its accessibility for seniors with mobility limitations or balance impairments. Standing upright for extended periods can be challenging for those with joint pain, fatigue, neuropathy, vertigo, or other age-related issues. Getting down onto the floor is an additional obstacle.

Chair-based stretches eliminate these barriers by safely allowing exercises to be performed from a stable, supported seated position. All stretches are done at chair height, reducing standing for long periods or transitioning to the mat. It opens up flexibility training to seniors who otherwise struggle with standing or lying positions.

Examples of conditions where chair stretching improves accessibility include:

- **Arthritis** - Joint inflammation and stiffness, especially in the knees or hips, can make standing difficult. Chair stretches relieve pain and improve mobility.

- **Low back pain** - Poor spinal flexion makes toe touches challenging. Seated rotation and side bends are less stressful.

- **Post-surgery** - Stretching while seated allows gentle movement after hip or knee replacements while avoiding standing.

- **Neuropathy** - Numbness or tingling in the feet reduces floor exercise stability. A chair provides support.

- **Reduced endurance** - Sitting to stretch combats fatigue and shortness of breath seniors might experience with upright exercise.

- **Dizziness** - Stretches like seated twists avoid position changes that can trigger lightheadedness in seniors.

- **Walker or Cane users** - Upper body stretches are easily done while seated with mobility aids safely nearby.

Chair stretching ensures seniors of all activity levels can safely perform a range of motion exercises. The stable seated position accommodates limitations while progressively building flexibility at an appropriate pace.

2. Comfort

Another advantage of chair stretching is the added comfort it provides seniors who struggle with certain movements and positions. The cushioned, supported seat reduces strain on the lower body. Stretches can be pain-free by adapting movements to avoid aggravated or painful joints.

Here are examples of how chair stretching offers comfort:

- A padded chair seat reduces pressure on the hips, knees, and back rather than standing the entire time.

- The chair provides lumbar support during spine and torso stretches.

- Armrests offer stabilization for safety and security.

- Stretches can be modified around knee or hip replacements by avoiding certain angles.

- Sitting avoids weight and pressure on sensitive joints, like arthritic knees or ankles.

- Choices of various stretches mean the painful ones can be avoided.

- Milder range of motion is possible by not forcing end ranges.

Chair stretching allows supportive aids like braces or splints to be comfortably worn during exercise. The ease, security, and support of performing stretches from a chair results in a joint-friendly flexibility regimen.

3. Strength Building

While chair stretches are focused on enhancing the range of motion, they also provide strength-building benefits. Specific seated stretches incorporate gentle muscle activation against gravity or resistance, improving coordination, endurance, and function.

Here are examples of strength gains:

- Arm raises strengthen the shoulders and upper back.

- Rotating and stretching the neck engages supportive cervical muscles.

- Lifting each leg activates the hip flexors and quadriceps.

- Plantar flexion and pointing the foot stimulate the calf muscles.

- Pressing the hands together adds effort to chest and shoulder stretches.

- Controlled twisting engages the core abdominal muscles.

Seniors should focus on the proper form by keeping the movements slow, smooth, and controlled. Avoid momentum or bouncing, which can strain muscles.

Chair stretches provide a mild strength training effect when done correctly. This helps maintain muscle tone and function essential for mobility. Flexibility and gentle strengthening make chair stretching a comprehensive exercise routine.

4. Safety

Chair stretching allows seniors to improve flexibility from a chair's safe, stable position. This minimizes the risk of falls or instability that can occur with standing or floor exercises. The chair supports and assists when lowering into and standing up from seated stretches.

Here are ways chair stretching enhances safety:

- A sturdy chair base prevents tipping or sliding.

- Seat support aids sitting down and standing up.

- Proximity to the chair assists equilibrium during balance-challenging stretches.

- Armrests offer added stability if unsteady or dizzy.

- Lower risk of strains due to overextending than standing positions.

- Falls are avoided since exercises are performed seated.

- Stretches can be performed conservatively within a safe range of motion.

For those recovering from recent falls or injuries, chair stretching provides secure rehabilitation before attempting riskier positions. Under guidance, chair stretches can improve mobility following hip fractures, knee operations, and low back procedures.

Chair-based stretches should be done regularly to gain full benefits. Integrate them throughout your day, while watching TV, at your desk, or during short breaks. Making seated stretches a daily habit improves flexibility, eases discomfort, and enhances well-being. Despite mobility or balance challenges, these exercises empower seniors to maintain an active, fulfilling lifestyle.

Chapter 8: Yoga for Seniors

Yoga uniquely benefits seniors by boosting flexibility, balance, strength, and mental wellness. Although it may seem intimidating initially, yoga can be adapted through senior-friendly routines that safely enhance mobility and vitality.

Introduction to Senior-Friendly Yoga

Yoga combines physical postures, breathing, and meditation to promote well-being. Senior-friendly yoga adapts this practice to meet older adults' needs. Here are essential yoga poses suitable for seniors:

Poses and Sequences Suitable for Seniors

1. Chair Yoga:

Chair yoga adapts traditional yoga poses using a chair, making them accessible for seniors with limited mobility. A stable chair allows users to perform poses safely while seated. Chair yoga poses include:

- **Seated Mountain Pose** - Sit tall, feet grounded, and sweep arms up alongside the ears with palms together. Improves spine alignment and shoulder flexibility.

- **Seated Twist** - Feet on the floor, twist the torso using core strength to place a hand on the opposite knee. Opens hips and shoulders and increases spinal mobility.

- **Seated Cat and Cow** - Arch and round spine while seated. Warms up the back and improves spinal flexibility.

- **Forward Fold** - Hinge at the hips and extend the arms forward with a flat back. Stretches hamstrings and the lower back.

- **Eagle Arms** - Cross one arm under the other, wrapping the arms together in front. Stretches upper back and shoulders.

- **Ankle Stretches** - Rotate ankles and flex and point the feet while seated. Increases ankle flexibility and circulation.

- **Leg Raises** - Extend one leg straight and raise off the chair while flexing the foot. Strengthens thighs and improves balance.

- **Spinal Twist** - Cross the leg over the opposite knee, and use your core to twist the torso. Therapeutic for lower back pain and stiffness.

- **Neck Stretches** - Tilt the neck gently from side to side. Relieves neck tension.

- **Figure Four Stretch** - Cross the ankle over the opposite knee and fold forward. Opens the hips.

Chair yoga allows users to perform seated postures with proper alignment while enjoying yoga's benefits. The stable base makes balance and coordination less demanding, while the armrests provide support as needed. Chair yoga enables those with mobility restrictions to improve flexibility safely.

2. Mountain Pose (Tadasana):

The mountain pose is a foundational standing posture that improves balance, posture, and concentration:

1. Stand with your big toes touching and heels slightly apart to ground the feet. Engage your leg muscles.

2. Lift the kneecaps and firm the thighs. Engage your core.

3. Inhale and sweep arms up alongside ears with palms together. Straighten the elbows.

4. Gaze straight ahead. Elongate the spine from the tailbone through the crown of the head.

5. Hold the pose for 5-8 breaths, focusing on steady breathing.

Benefits include:

- Improves posture and alignment of the spine, shoulders, and neck.

- Engages the leg and core muscles and increases lower body strength.

- Challenges balance and concentration.

- Opens the chest and shoulders and stretches the upper body.

- Teaches a foundation for other standing poses, establishing a proper form.

Use a wall or chair for support if needed. Modify the pose with your hands on the hips if raising the arms overhead is difficult.

3. Tree Pose (Vrksasana):

The tree pose challenges balance and stimulates concentration:

1. Shift your weight to the left leg. Bend the right knee and place the right foot on the left inner thigh.

2. Press the right foot firmly into the thigh. Avoid resting the foot on the knee joint.

3. Place your hands in a prayer position at the heart center or reach the arms overhead.

4. Gaze at a fixed point to help balance. Hold for 30-60 seconds.

5. Repeat on the other side, placing the left foot against the right inner thigh.

Benefits include:

- Improves coordination, balance, and concentration.

- Strengthens the legs, ankles, and core.

- Increases focus and awareness.

- Therapeutic for relieving sciatica.

Use a wall or chair for hand support if needed. Modify the pose by placing the foot against the calf instead of the thigh if hamstring flexibility is limited.

4. Downward-Facing Dog (Adho Mukha Svanasana):

Downward dog provides a full body stretch while building strength:

1. From the tabletop position, tuck your toes under and lift the hips up and back.

2. Press your hands firmly down, and straighten the arms and legs. Form an inverted V shape.

3. With the feet hip-width apart and the heels reaching toward the floor, gently straighten your knees.

4. Hold for 30-60 seconds, breathing deeply.

Benefits include:

- Stretches the hamstrings, calves, hips, and shoulders.

- Strengthens arms and legs.

- Improves posture.

- Provides mild inversion and increases spinal traction and extension.

Use bent knees to modify the pose. Avoid this pose if high blood pressure is a concern.

5. Child's Pose (Balasana):

The child's pose releases tension and gently stretches the lower back:

1. From all fours, bring your big toes together, knees wide apart.

2. Exhale and sit the hips back over the heels, lowering the torso between the thighs.

3. The forehead rests on the floor. Reach the arms forward or rest them alongside the body.

4. Hold the pose for 30-60 seconds, breathing deeply.

Benefits include:

- Stretches the lower back, hips, and thighs.

- Reduces stress and fatigue and calms the mind.

- Gently stimulates digestive organs.

- Provides mild inversion and decompresses the spine.

Use a bolster under the forehead for support if the floor is too far. The arm position can be varied for comfort. Keep knees separated to avoid hip strain.

6. Corpse Pose (Savasana):

Corpse pose offers complete relaxation and restoration:

1. Lay on your back and ensure that your legs are spread, relaxing your toes.

2. Place your arms at your side, make sure your palms are upwards.

3. Close your eyes and breathe deeply through the nose.

4. Scan and relax each body part methodically from the toes to the head.

5. Hold for 5-10 minutes.

Benefits include:

- Promotes mental clarity and relaxation.

- Reduces stress, anxiety, fatigue, and headache.

- Lowers blood pressure and the resting heart rate.

- Prepares the body for meditation and deep sleep.

- Integrates benefits of yoga practice.

Support the head, knees, or back with bolsters, blankets, or blocks if needed. Savasana restores the mind and body, making it an essential concluding pose.

These 6 poses provide a sampling of yoga's many benefits for seniors. When appropriately modified, yoga can be accessible and enjoyable for practitioners of all ability levels. A balanced yoga practice improves holistic well-being in the second half of life.

How Yoga Can Improve Flexibility and Balance

Yoga is an ancient Indian practice that's been around for thousands of years. The Sanskrit word "yoga" means to join or unite, which is precisely what yoga aims for — to unite your mind, body, and spirit through poses, breathing techniques, and meditation.

Yoga can help improve health in many ways for older adults. Two significant benefits are better flexibility and balance. The gentle stretching and positioning in the poses help increase the range of motion in your joints and lengthen muscles. Yoga strengthens your core and improves stability, leading to better balance and fewer falls.

1. How Yoga Boosts Flexibility

As you get on in years, it's common for flexibility to decrease. Your joints lose their range of motion, the muscles get tighter, and the tissues get less elastic. Regularly practicing yoga can help counteract these changes by moving your body through full ranges of motion.

Each yoga pose stretches different muscle groups and joints. For example, sitting cross-legged stretches your hips, knees, and ankles. Standing poses like Warrior I and II work your hips, shoulders, and legs. Seated forward folds lengthen your spine and the backs of your legs. As your body becomes more flexible, you can perform deeper into the poses, increasing flexibility even more.

Yoga promotes mind-body awareness. Being present as you stretch allows you to slowly ease into poses at your own pace. Focusing on steady, mindful breathing, you can hold poses longer, giving your muscles and tissues more time to relax and release. This restores mobility to your joints and improves overall flexibility.

Some yoga poses that are especially good for boosting flexibility include:

- **Cat and Cow** - Gently flexes and extends the spine. Great for spinal flexibility.

- **Downward Dog** - Stretches hips, hamstrings, calves, shoulders and spine.

- **Wide-Legged Forward Fold** - Lengthens hamstrings and inner thighs.

- **Bridge Pose** - Strengthens the back while opening the chest and hips.

- **Butterfly** - Stretches inner thighs and groin.

- **Seated Spinal Twist** - Rotates spine for a greater range of motion.

Focusing on poses that gently open you up rather than intensely stretching is important. Being mindful and moving slowly through each pose allows the muscles to relax into deeper flexibility. Practicing patiently, without forcing progress, keeps yoga therapeutic and helps your body become suppler over time.

2. Enhancing Balance through Yoga

As you get older, your balance declines. Many factors contribute to poorer stability, including weaker muscles, impaired vision or inner ear function, neurological changes, and medication side effects. Falls become increasingly common as balance diminishes with age, so practicing yoga can help improve stability and prevent falls.

Yoga strengthens the muscles for balance, like the ankles, legs, hips, abdomen, and back. Standing poses, like Tree Pose and Warrior III, require coordination to stabilize the body. Moving between standing and seated poses develops transitional balance. Yoga improves proprioception - awareness of the body's position in space - for better balance.

Additionally, focused breathing and concentration while holding poses train seniors to tune into the body's subtle sensations. This mental focus and physical strength gain results in enhanced mind-body connection for improved balance and coordination.

Poses that specifically target balance include:

- **Tree Pose** - Standing on one leg strengthens the legs while improving focus.

- **Eagle Pose** - Challenges balance by crossing the legs and arms.

- **Dancer's Pose** - Requires balance to grasp the foot behind you.

- **Chair Pose** - Strengthens the legs while training balance.

- **Warrior III** - Works balance by extending one leg straight back.

- **Crescent Lunge** - Stability is required to power the front leg.

Practicing these yoga poses reduces the risk of falling. However, seniors new to yoga should always practice near a wall, chair, or counter for hand support to avoid injury if balance wavers. As core strength and stability improve, balancing poses can be practiced independently.

Get Started Slowly and Safely

For seniors new to yoga, starting a routine safely and gradually is essential. Strenuous yoga should be avoided. Instead, look for classes described as senior yoga, gentle yoga, or restorative yoga.

Before beginning a yoga practice, seniors should consult their doctor, especially those with injuries, chronic conditions, or balance impairments. Make the instructor aware of limitations or concerns before class. Work closely with the teacher to modify poses as needed. Never force the body into uncomfortable positions.

Build up yoga sessions slowly. Begin with just 10-15 minutes once or twice a week. Pause between poses frequently. Allow the body to warm up thoroughly before deeper stretching. Use props like blocks and straps to ease into poses more gently. Focus on comfortable postures rather than perfect alignment and gradually increase the practice duration and intensity over several weeks.

Enjoying the benefits of yoga requires consistency. But it's important not to overexert - know when to take breaks to avoid soreness or fatigue. Stay hydrated before, during, and after yoga. Listen to your body and be cautious as you increase flexibility.

While yoga studios offer guidance and social interaction, at-home practices allow seniors to go at their own pace. Follow with yoga videos for seniors from trusted sources. Seek out instructors with experience in adapting poses for less mobile bodies. Always allow time after class for relaxation.

Yoga Is More Than Just Physical

While yoga offers clear physical benefits, like improved flexibility and balance, it provides much more. Yoga's meditative nature brings mental and emotional well-being. The practice encourages seniors to clear their minds, relax, and focus on the present. Moving through sequences with controlled breathing induces the "relaxation response" to counter everyday stress. Yoga provides an outlet for seniors to move comfortably and confidently.

Regular yoga practice allows seniors to tune into their bodies and become more in touch with their needs and abilities. Yoga helps relieve joint pain and stiffness that may seem normal and inevitable. Deep breathing during yoga boosts energy and fights fatigue. Seniors often notice improved sleep and a calmer overall state of mind.

The social interactions provided by yoga classes benefit emotional health. Practicing in a group setting combats isolation and forges connections. Yoga gives seniors a sense of community and support. Lifelong learning is fostered by acquiring new skills and continuously evolving a yoga practice.

Yoga enables seniors to move more freely and live more vibrantly. While yoga has roots in spiritual transcendence, the benefits from a consistent practice are deeply tangible. Often, seniors who embrace yoga describe gains that transform their daily lives, such as:

- Greater ease of movement and less pain when walking, bending, or doing chores.

- Increased independence, caring for themselves, and confidence in living alone.

- Less fear and anxiety, and improved relaxation.

- Feeling energized, strong, optimistic, and more "like myself" again.

- Deeper sleep and mental focus.

- Enjoyment, fulfillment, and social connections.

By nourishing the body and soul, seniors can experience these life-enhancing rewards. They can participate in activities they love with greater comfort, freedom, and pleasure. Yoga enables aging with strength, stability, and grace.

Chapter 9: Pilates for Seniors

Pilates is a gentle, low-impact exercise that strengthens your core, increases flexibility, and improves body awareness. It's great for seniors aiming to maintain physical health and mobility. This chapter introduces senior-friendly Pilates, its benefits, and mat exercises to boost your strength and flexibility.

Overview of Pilates for Seniors

Pilates is a unique exercise originally developed by a German man, Joseph Pilates, in the early 20th century. After moving to England in the 1910s, Pilates refined controlled and precise movements to strengthen the body from the inside out. Over the next few decades, Pilates continued developing his revolutionary system of mind-body exercise.

By the 1960s, his techniques had gained popularity around the world. Today, Pilates is practiced by millions of people and has become one of the most popular low-impact exercises. For seniors, Pilates offers a safe yet challenging way to build core strength, improve flexibility, and enhance mental clarity.

Joseph Pilates believed strongly in the mind-body connection. All his techniques emphasize mental focus, proper breathing, and smooth, deliberate movements. "Contrology," as he initially called his method, targets the deep abdomen and back muscles that comprise the body's core.

Pilates realized that strengthening these core muscles could improve overall strength and coordination throughout the entire body. A strong powerhouse, or core, also corrects postural imbalances, eases back pain, and stabilizes the spine.

Another key principle of Pilates is precision. Each exercise follows a strict sequence of motions to elongate, strengthen, and balance the body. Pilates movements promote grace, flexibility, and economy of motion when performed with control. Breath is also integral to Pilates. Special breathing patterns help energize the body, oxygenate the blood, and focus intention.

Over the decades, Joseph Pilates' original 34 mat exercises have expanded into a comprehensive system practiced on mats and specialized equipment. While the repertoire has grown, the principles of core strength, precision, flow, and breath remain the foundation. For aging individuals hoping to retain (or regain) strength, mobility, and balance, Pilates techniques specifically for seniors can offer incredible benefits.

Several key advantages make Pilates an excellent exercise for older adults. Some of the main benefits of a Pilates practice for seniors include:

1. **Core Strength:**

The core is the muscles in the trunk and pelvis regions - abdominals, lower back, hips, glutes, and deep spinal muscles. Weak core muscles can cause poor posture, instability, and back pain. Many daily activities require core strength to perform basic functional movements like getting up from a chair. A strong core is the foundation for every exercise in Pilates.

By activating deep abdominal muscles, Pilates boosts core fitness, which translates to better balance, mobility, and injury prevention. Specific Pilates movements like "hundreds," crunches, and leg pull-downs target the abdominal muscles.

Other exercises called "swimming" and "superman" strengthen lower back muscles. Working the core also fosters greater body awareness. Seniors with improved core fitness have increased stability and control over their movements. A strong core empowers seniors to perform daily activities and confidently live actively.

2. Flexibility:

As you age, the body's tissues lose elasticity. Muscles and joints become stiffer, and the range of motion decreases. Practicing Pilates enhances flexibility, which is crucial for seniors' mobility. Proper stretching is incorporated into Pilates routines, and exercises like forward bends, spinal twists, and shoulder rolls lengthen tight muscles.

Other poses focus on joint mobility by taking them through complete ranges of motion. For example, circling the ankles, wrists, and shoulders lubricates joints. Dynamic sequences that move from flexion to extension increase overall limberness. Combining strengthening with stretching, Pilates creates supple, elastic muscles that move freely through their full range.

Seniors who commit to regular Pilates practice increase joint mobility and flexibility. They find everyday motions like looking over the shoulder, reaching down, or stepping high more manageable. Boosting flexibility allows seniors to tie shoes, garden, golf, and complete the activities they love with greater comfort.

3. Low-Impact:

High-impact exercises like running can aggravate joint pain and cause injuries for aging bodies. But Pilates provides a gentle strength-building alternative that is easy on the joints. Pilates' smooth, controlled movements do not pound the joints, and by engaging the deep core muscles, pressure on the spine and limbs is reduced.

Pilates exercises can be done standing, seated, or lying down - accommodating physical limitations. No jumping or high-velocity motions are involved. The pace is low to moderate and adaptable for individual needs.

Additionally, Pilates improves alignment and corrects muscle imbalances, leading to joint wear and tear. Developing core strength takes the pressure off the neck, knees, and back.

Overall, Pilates allows seniors to become stronger and more flexible while avoiding further joint damage. Even those with arthritis and injuries can practice Pilates safely. By protecting the joints and reducing pain, seniors' mobility and quality of life improve.

4. Mental Clarity:

There is a meditative quality to Pilates' focused movements and breathwork. Performing the sequences requires concentration and precision, demanding mental engagement and improving cognitive skills like memory, coordination, and reaction time. The mind-body connection is continually fostered.

Additionally, the emphasis on full, deep breathing has calming effects. Inhaling and exhaling consciously while moving reduces anxiety and stress. Endorphins released during Pilates provide mood-boosting benefits.

Overall, the mental stamina, stress relief, and biofeedback gained from Pilates keeps the mind sharper and more positive. Seniors derive a sense of accomplishment from mastering the exercises and seeing their physical abilities improve - enhancing self-confidence and vitality. For these reasons, many seniors find their regular Pilates routines therapeutic and stimulating.

Mat-Based Exercises for Core Strength and Flexibility

To enjoy the benefits of Pilates safely and effectively, seniors should consider the following:

- **Consult your doctor** - Make sure Pilates is appropriate, especially if you have medical issues, injuries, or balance problems. Inform your instructor.

- **Start slowly** - Allow time to learn proper form and build endurance. Begin with only 10-15 minutes, 1-2 times a week.

- **Focus on quality** - Precision is crucial in Pilates. Move slowly and control each motion. Proper form prevents injury.

- **Use modifications** - Any exercise can be adapted with props like cushions or chairs. Know your limits.

- **Work with experience** - Find an instructor educated in Pilates for seniors and adult beginners. Private or small group classes are ideal.

- **Listen to your body** - Pilates should never cause pain. Stop uncomfortable moves and rest when needed.

- **Practice patience** - Progress will come with consistency. Allow the muscles time to strengthen and the joints to become more flexible.

Pilates should never be strained. Seniors find Pilates rewarding and invigorating at any age or ability level when performed correctly. A customized Pilates routine offers seniors a path to maintaining and improving physical and mental fitness.

Here are five beginner Pilates mat exercises tailored specifically for seniors:

1. The Hundred

The Hundred is a classic Pilates abdominal exercise that builds core endurance while practicing breath control.

1. Lay on your mat on your back and extend your legs. Arms rest by your sides.

2. Inhale as you raise yourself starting from the heads all the way down to your shoulders.

3. Raise both arms straight up toward the ceiling with palms down.

4. As you exhale, briskly pump your arms up and down about 6-8 inches, keeping the movement controlled.

5. Inhale and exhale through your nose for 5 breath cycles as you continue pumping your arms.

6. Each set of 5 inhales and exhales counts as one repetition. Complete a total of 10 repetitions, or "100" breaths.

7. Keep your neck and shoulders relaxed, supporting your upper body with your core as you pump your arms.

8. If needed, bend your knees or place your feet flat on the floor to support the lower back.

9. Rest and repeat for 1-3 sets. Build your endurance over time.

This energizing hundred sequence strengthens the abdominal muscles while stabilizing the back. It improves core stamina, which is essential for balance and mobility and preventing injury from falls. The controlled breathing focus helps seniors concentrate and quieten their mental chatter.

2. Leg Circles

Leg Circles target the hips' deep muscles and inner thighs. Circumducting the legs in full ranges of motion increases hip joint flexibility.

1. Lie on your back with both legs fully extended. Arms relax on the floor by your sides.

2. First, take a deep breath in, then as you release it, raise your left leg while keeping the right stationary.

3. Inhale and trace a small circle with your right foot, rotating at the hip. Complete 5-10 circles clockwise.

4. Reverse the direction to complete 5-10 circles counter-clockwise. Maintain stability in your torso and stationary left leg.

5. Lower your right leg back down next to the left. Repeat the full circle sequence with the left leg lifting and circling.

6. Continue alternating legs for 5-10 circles in each direction, on each side.

7. Gradually make the circles bigger over time, but control the motion using the deep hip rotators.

8. Rest briefly between sides to reset.

The hip mobility and core control required during Leg Circles increases seniors' flexibility, coordination, and balance. It makes everyday activities like getting dressed or stepping over obstacles safer and easier.

3. Bridging

Bridging strengthens the glutes, hamstrings, and core muscles for improved stability.

1. Lie on your back with the knees bent at 90 degrees, feet flat on the floor about hip-width apart. Arms rest on the floor by your sides.

2. Inhale to engage your core, then exhale as you tilt your pelvis and lift your hips off the mat. Press evenly through your heels to straighten your spine into a diagonal line.

3. Take a deep breath in, then let it out when you are lowering your hips. Keep your core engaged throughout.

4. Repeat for 5-10 bridges, building the repetitions over time. Move slowly and steadily.

5. For added difficulty, raise one leg straight as you lift into the Bridge. Alternate legs.

6. Rest briefly between Bridges.

Bridging strengthens the glutes and hamstrings, which stabilizes the hips and knees. The exercise firms up abdominal muscles when done with proper pelvic placement. Regular Bridging gives seniors greater strength and control for daily functions like standing up, walking, bending, and balancing.

4. Swimming

Swimming mimics the crawl stroke to work the core muscles of the back and abdomen.

1. Lie on your stomach with your legs extended straight behind you and the tops of your feet on the floor. Stretch your arms overhead on the mat with palms down.

2. Inhale to prepare. As you exhale, simultaneously raise your right arm and left leg several inches off the floor.

3. Inhale as you lower your right arm and left leg.

4. Exhale, lifting your left arm and right leg. Continue alternating sides steadily for 10-20 repetitions.

5. Keep your head, neck, and hips square and stable. Avoid arching your back.

6. Move smoothly between the sides like a swimming stroke. Control each lift and lowering.

7. Rest briefly, then repeat for 1-2 sets.

The coordination required in Swimming strengthens muscles deep in the spine, improving spinal alignment. Raising the arms and legs against gravity also firms the back, shoulders, glutes, and hamstrings. Overall, core control gets a great workout with this Pilates move.

5. Seated Forward Bend

The Seated Forward Bend is a wonderful hip and hamstring stretch.

1. Sit tall on your mat with your legs extended in front of you. Feet flexed.

2. Inhale and sweep your arms overhead. Feel the stretch through your sides.

3. Exhale and hinge forward from your hips, reaching your arms toward your feet. Let your head and neck relax.

4. Hold the stretch for 15-30 seconds using deep belly breaths. Reach your hands toward your ankles if you cannot touch your toes.

5. Inhale back to the center when ready, lifting through the spine to return upright.

6. Repeat 2-3 times, going only as far forward as comfortable for your flexibility.

The Seated Forward Bend improves mobility in the hips and hamstrings. It allows seniors to bend down to pick things up or step into a car more comfortably and efficiently.

As you continue learning these five introductory mat exercises, focus on moving slowly and gently. Proper form and breath control prevent injury and make Pilates more effective. Be patient, building reps and range of motion over time. With consistent Pilates practice, seniors gain stronger cores, looser joints, balanced muscles, and renewed energy.

Adaptations for Seniors with Different Fitness Levels

One of Pilates' great benefits for seniors is that it can be adapted and modified to suit all fitness levels. While Pilates strengthens the core, improves flexibility, and challenges balance and coordination, it is a customizable practice. Seniors who are only starting can make exercises easier, while more active seniors have many options to intensify their routines. With simple modifications using props or adjustments to the range of motion, seniors at all activity levels can find an appropriate Pilates routine.

For Beginner Seniors:

Seniors who are new to exercise or have not been active for some time should start Pilates at a basic level. Beginner seniors may need to modify exercises by:

- **Reducing range of motion** - Only move through comfortable ranges, avoiding strain or discomfort. Slowly work toward larger movements.

- **Fewer repetitions** - Start with 5-10 reps of a movement and gradually build up to higher repetitions as your strength increases.

- **Slower pace** - Move through exercises slowly and with complete control over the motion. Avoid quick or jerky movements.

- **More rest** - Take breaks between exercises and allow plenty of time for the body to recover after a session.

- **Use of props** - Cushions, blocks, or chairs can provide extra support and stability when needed.

Examples of how to modify Pilates for less conditioned seniors include:

- Keeping one foot on the floor during leg lifts or circles.

- Holding onto a chair when balancing to avoid falls.

- Only raising the torso halfway in abdominal crunches.

- Sitting upright vs. lying flat for comfort.

- Keeping the range of motion small in stretches.

The aim for Pilates beginners is to build a foundation slowly. Over several weeks, the body adapts, becoming stronger and more flexible. Seniors gain confidence and can gradually progress to more advanced moves with consistent practice at a manageable level.

For Active or Fit Seniors:

For seniors accustomed to regular exercise, Pilates can be performed at a more challenging level:

- **Full range of motion** - Extend movements to increase intensity through the complete joint range.

- **Added resistance** - Use light hand weights or resistance bands to strengthen moves.

- **Dynamic transitions** - Flow smoothly from one exercise to the next to elevate heart rate.

- **Increased repetitions** - Build muscular endurance with higher repetition sets.

- **Sustained holds** - Isometrically holds a challenging position like a plank for an extended time.

- **One-leg variations** - Perform lifts, circles, or balances on one leg to increase difficulty.

- **Eye gaze** - Fix your eyes straight ahead during balance poses rather than looking down.

Modifications to make Pilates harder include:

- Straight leg raises aimed at a 45-degree angle.

- Roll-up with straight legs vs. bent knees.

- Holding the side plank for 30-60 seconds before lowering.

- Raising arms overhead during bridges for counterbalance.

- A higher number of upper body reps like chest flys or swimming.

Adding intensity allows fitter seniors to keep progressing. However, maintaining control and proper form with every motion is critical. Moving faster through exercises is not advised, as this increases injury risk. The focus should remain on quality movement over quantity. Pilates can be made more difficult while being gentle on the joints and safe for active seniors.

Adapting Pilates for Special Health Conditions:

Extra caution is required for some health conditions like osteoporosis, joint replacement, or cardiac issues. Specific movements must be avoided, and close guidance from an experienced Pilates instructor is recommended. Suggestions include:

1. **Osteoporosis:**

   - Avoid spinal twists and forward bends that compress vertebrae.

   - Use a small range of motion and very light resistance.

   - Modify exercises to be performed seated if needed.

2. **Joint Replacement:**

   - Avoid weight-bearing on affected joints if recommended by the surgeon.

   - Reduce the range of motion to remain comfortable.

- Build strength gradually around surgical sites.

3. Cardiac Issues:

- Check with your doctor for exercise clearance.

- Start with shorter, gentle sessions.

- Modify exercises to be performed sitting or lying down.

- Monitor heart rate and breathing closely.

The great thing about Pilates is that almost anyone can participate safely with adaptive equipment like chairs or modifications to reduce weight-bearing. Seniors with health conditions should consult their doctor and Pilates instructor closely to ensure exercises are appropriate.

The Benefits of Adapted Pilates for Seniors

The ability to modify Pilates for all senior fitness levels is wonderful. Whether new to exercise or accustomed to regular workouts, seniors can find the right challenge. Pilates can be made easier or more intense as needed.

Adapted Pilates allows seniors to keep progressing at their own pace. Maintaining appropriate alignment and control is fundamental to every properly modified exercise. Hence, Pilates is rewarding for all under guidance from instructors experienced with seniors.

Through regular practice of adapted Pilates, seniors become stronger, more flexible, and stable - improving mobility, independence, and vitality.

Chapter 10: Resistance Band Exercises for Seniors

Resistance bands are super versatile exercise tools that help older adults improve strength, balance, and flexibility. They give resistance to make your muscles work hard without heavy weights or high-impact moves. So bands are a gentle way to strength train for folks at any fitness level. This chapter discusses resistance band exercises tailored for seniors. It talks about the benefits of regularly exercising with resistance bands. They're a safe, low-impact way to gain strength and stability as you age.

Benefits of Resistance Band Exercises for Seniors

Resistance band workouts offer seniors an extremely effective yet low-impact way to improve overall fitness. They are large elastic bands available in various resistance levels and sizes. When stretched, they resist movements, helping build strength through the range of motion. Some major benefits include:

1. **Low Impact:**

As you age, your joints become increasingly vulnerable to arthritis and injury. High-impact activities like running can aggravate joint pain and damage the cartilage. But resistance band training offers seniors a comfortably low-impact alternative. The elastic bands provide resistance to challenge the muscles gently, avoiding jarring movements that can lead to joint issues.

Resistance band exercises are performed slowly and controlled rather than with momentum or ballistic motions that may strain the joints. The elasticity absorbs shock for the knees, hips, and other vulnerable joints, making resistance bands preferable for those with arthritis, injuries, or pre-existing joint problems.

Even vigorous resistance band routines allow seniors to strengthen their bodies without added joint pain and inflammation. Resistance bands enable safe, effective training to preserve bone density, muscle mass, and mobility.

2. Versatility:

One of the most significant aspects of resistance bands is their versatility for exercising all the major muscle groups. The bands come in a wide range of resistance levels, so seniors can start with light bands and gradually progress to more intense resistance as their strength improves. The bands can be anchored in multiple positions to target different muscles. They are tremendously portable, allowing seniors to exercise at home or on the go. Examples of total-body resistance band exercises include:

Upper Body:

- Bicep curls

- Overhead tricep extensions.

- Shoulder presses

- Chest flys

- Reverse flys for the back.

- Seated rows

Lower Body:

- Squats

- Lateral walks

- Standing leg abductions.

- Seated knee extensions.

- Donkey kicks for glutes.

- Inner and outer thigh work.

Core:

- Standing torso twists.

- Seated Russian twists.

- Bent-over back extensions.

- Side bends

- Front and lateral plank walks.

The wide range of full-body movements possible with resistance bands allows seniors to target any muscle group. Routines can be customized to specific goals like building upper body strength for daily tasks or improving core stability for better balance. Having so many exercise options keeps resistance band workouts stimulating.

3. Strength and Endurance:

Maintaining muscular fitness is crucial for seniors' mobility, daily functioning, and independence. Strength declines with age as muscle fibers atrophy due to inactivity. This loss of lean muscle mass is called sarcopenia. However, research shows resistance training can help counteract this natural decline.

Resistance bands provide sufficient overload on the muscles to promote gains in both strength and muscular endurance. The continuous tension of the stretched bands throughout a movement strengthens muscles in all motion angles, leading to notable increases in the force muscles can exert. Higher rep sets with lighter resistance build endurance for extended daily tasks.

Increased strength and stamina make activities like lifting heavy objects, yard work, climbing stairs, and extended shopping trips more manageable. Only 10-20 minutes of resistance band training 2-3 times a week can benefit seniors' daily lifestyles.

4. Improved Balance:

As seniors age, balance and stability commonly decline. Contributing factors include muscle loss, slower reflexes, declining vision, and poor proprioception. Improving balance helps prevent falls, a leading cause of hospitalization and disability for older adults.

Many resistance band exercises train the body's balance and stabilization systems simultaneously as strength is gained. Moves like standing rows, overhead presses, and side leg lifts require the body to stabilize against the band's resistance. Balancing on one foot when using bands improves control. Integrating focused balance training into band routines, like proprioceptive moves on a BOSU ball, can further improve stability.

Resistance band training strengthens the muscles essential for catching yourself before a fall. It equates to better daily function for seniors, whether walking on uneven surfaces, reaching on tiptoes, or getting in and out of a car.

5. Portability:

One reason resistance band training is so ideal for seniors is the convenience of using the bands anytime. Seniors don't need access to workout machines or free weights to reap the benefits of resistance training. Compact resistance bands are inexpensive and can be used almost anywhere. Seniors can efficiently perform full routines in the comfort of their homes without a gym membership.

Resistance band workouts are extremely portable when traveling or away from home. They take up minimal space when packed, and many hotels provide bands in fitness rooms. Simple resistance bands make it easy for seniors to maintain regular strength training routines while on vacation and away from typical exercise facilities.

At home, seniors may feel more motivated to work out in private than in a crowded gym setting, and the convenience eliminates transit time to a fitness center. The accessibility of home resistance band workouts removes many barriers to seniors staying active consistently.

Resistance Band Exercises for Seniors

Here are five foundational resistance band exercises ideal for seniors:

1. Bicep Curls:

Place the resistance band securely under both feet, positioning feet about hip-width apart. Grab one end of the band in each hand with palms facing forward.

1. Stand tall, engaging your core. Keeping your elbows close at your sides, slowly bend both elbows and curl your hands toward your shoulders to contract the biceps.

2. Focus on controlled motion and keep the shoulders down throughout the curl. Breathe out as you curl the band up.

3. Pause briefly at the top of the curl with the biceps fully contracted. Inhale as you slowly lower your arms back to the starting position.

4. Start with 10-15 controlled reps for 1-2 sets. Add more reps or sets as your strength increases.

5. Make it easier by choosing a lighter resistance band. Increase the intensity with a heavier resistance band when able.

6. You can alternate arms, performing one arm at a time. Or curl both arms simultaneously, depending on your ability.

The bicep curl strengthens the front upper arms - essential for lifting and carrying objects like groceries. Strong biceps facilitate pulling motions, like opening doors.

2. Leg Extensions:

1. Sit upright in a sturdy chair and securely loop one end of the resistance band around your right leg's ankle.

2. Hold the ends of the band firmly in each hand near your shoulders, elbows bent.

3. Keeping your ankle flexed, slowly extend your right leg directly out in front of you against the band's resistance.

4. Inhale as you extend your leg fully. Focus on using the quadriceps. Exhale slowly, bending the knee to return to the starting position.

5. Complete 10-15 controlled repetitions. Complete 2 sets on the right leg.

6. Switch the band to the left ankle and repeat for 2 sets on the left leg.

7. Increase the resistance band tension for more intensity when able. Decrease band tension if needed.

The leg extension strengthens the quadriceps muscles on the front of the thighs. Strong quads are needed for stability when walking, climbing stairs, standing from a chair, and many other daily activities.

3. Rowing Motion:

1. Sit tall on a chair with your feet flat on the floor about hip-width apart. Extend your arms toward the floor with palms facing each other.

2. Secure the center of the band under both feet. Then, grasp one band end in each hand.

3. Initiate the rowing motion by pulling your hands toward the side of your torso and squeezing your shoulder blades as you row.

4. Focus on squeezing the muscles between your shoulder blades as you pull your elbows back.

5. Inhale slowly as you straighten your arms back to the starting position.

6. Complete 10-15 controlled rows for 2 sets.

7. Increase resistance band tension over time to work the back muscles harder.

8. You can alternate the arms if needed to build unilateral upper back strength.

This rowing exercise strengthens the upper back while improving posture. Strong upper back musculature can alleviate neck, shoulder, and upper back pain.

4. Hip Abduction:

1. Start by standing behind a chair or counter, holding on for balance. Place the resistance band securely around both ankles.

2. Slowly lift your right leg straight out to the side against the band's resistance, moving from the hip. Keep left leg stable.

3. Inhale as you open the right hip and abduct your leg. Exhale slowly lowering your right leg but don't rest it on the floor.

4. Complete 10-15 controlled repetitions, keeping tension on the band at all times.

5. Complete 2 sets on the right side, then switch the band to the left ankle and repeat for 2 sets.

6. Increase the resistance band intensity over time to strengthen the hip abductors further.

7. Keep the hips square and the spine straight throughout the motion. Avoid leaning.

Strengthening the muscles that abduct the hips improves stability for walking, standing up from chairs, getting in and out of cars, and stepping over objects.

5. Standing Balance Exercise:

1. Secure one end of the resistance band under the ball of your right foot. Stand upright, holding the other end of the band in each hand by your sides. Engage your core.

2. Exhale as you slowly raise both arms straight out to your sides against the pull of the band. Pause for 1 second. This requires balance to resist tipping.

3. Inhale, bringing your arms slowly back to your sides. Repeat 10-15 times.

4. Complete 2-3 sets while balanced on your right leg, focusing on steady breath and a tight core.

5. Switch the band to left foot and complete 2-3 sets on the other side.

6. Increase the band's resistance level to make the balance challenge harder.

This total body balance exercise strengthens the legs while training stability and control. Enhancing balance helps prevent falls among seniors.

Safety Tips for Resistance Band Exercises

Resistance band workouts are incredibly beneficial strength training for seniors. The elastic bands provide gentle resistance to improve muscle strength, mobility, and stability.

However, seniors must perform resistance band exercises safely to gain the benefits while avoiding injury. Resistance training has immense health advantages if done correctly using appropriate precautions. Here are top tips to optimize safety and effectiveness when doing resistance band routines:

1. Choose the Right Resistance Level

Resistance bands come in a range of tension levels, from light resistance (often color-coded yellow or red) to heavy resistance (commonly black, silver, or green bands). Choosing a band that provides the proper resistance for your current strength and fitness is crucial. The band tension must challenge your muscles but not be so difficult you can't complete the full range of motion.

If you're new to resistance training, start with the lightest band. You should perform 8-15 reps of an exercise while maintaining good form. The band is too challenging if your motions become sloppy or uncontrolled. Conversely, if a band feels too easy and you can do over 15 reps perfectly, you need more resistance.

Build your strength over several weeks before moving to a more challenging resistance band. It's always better to start slow and light to master safe technique. Proper form should come before adding intensity.

Listen to your body's feedback as you progress through your resistance band workouts. Some indicators that you need a lighter band include:

- Inability to complete all the prescribed reps and sets.

- Muscle shaking when performing an exercise.

- Breaking proper form because the resistance is too heavy.

- Straining or discomfort in joints.

- Holding your breath during movements due to exertion.

- Dizziness or excessive fatigue after a resistance workout.

If you experience these warning signs, immediately switch to a lighter resistance band. Feeling some muscle fatigue is normal, but no exercise should be painful or dangerous.

Only increase band resistance when you can fully complete reps with proper form and control. Choosing bands that appropriately match your abilities will keep resistance training safe, effective, and enjoyable.

2. Maintain Proper Form and Technique

In addition to the right resistance level, practicing perfect exercise techniques is vital for safety with resistance bands. Proper alignment protects the joints by keeping them stabilized and avoiding overstretching. Smooth, controlled motions prevent excessive strain or unexpected movements that can cause injury, especially to vulnerable senior joints.

Learning the ideal technique for every exercise takes practice and patience. It's smart to start by mastering form with lightweight resistance, allowing you to focus on precision. Avoid "cheating" or using momentum to complete motions with heavier resistance than you can safely handle.

Some key form tips include:

- Keep movements slow and steady. Avoid jerking or rapid motions.

- Maintain a strong yet relaxed posture. Avoid locking joints.

- Keep abdominal muscles engaged for a stable core throughout.

- Breathe naturally. Don't hold your breath during exertion.

- Keep wrists neutral rather than flexed or extended.

- Ensure full ranges of motion with control. No partial reps.

- Focus on proper muscle group initiation.

- Squeeze targeted muscles at the peak contraction point.

- Don't hyperextend joints or round the back.

When first getting started, having a trainer or physical therapist instruct you on the ideal technique for resistance band exercises is extremely helpful. They can guide body positioning, muscle engagement, and motion efficiency. Pay close attention to maintaining proper alignment and control throughout every movement if exercising at home alone. Use mirrors to self-correct if possible. Never sacrifice safe form to perform more reps or use a heavier resistance band. Patience and precision prevent injury.

3. Remember to Breathe Properly

It's common for people to hold their breath or irregularly breathe when exerting force against resistance. However, holding your breath can spike blood pressure to unsafe levels. Breathing normally and continuously throughout resistance band exercises is necessary to provide the working muscles with adequate oxygen. Not properly breathing leads to early fatigue since oxygen powers muscular performance.

Fully inhale and exhale as you contract and release the muscles during each resistance band motion. Time your breathing with your pace of movement. Generally, inhale as muscles lengthen and prepare to engage, then exhale as you contract the muscles against the resistance. Keep a steady, controlled breath pattern even as you fatigue.

If you cannot maintain normal breathing, it's a sign to reduce the exercise intensity. Proper breathing technique during resistance training helps relax the mind and body between exercises. Don't disregard breathing fundamentals when focusing on muscle movements. Oxygen is fuel for your workout and essential for safety.

4. Seek Professional Guidance When Needed

For seniors who are entirely new to resistance training or have pre-existing health concerns, seeking guidance from a fitness professional is highly recommended. Experienced trainers can teach proper technique, provide exercise modifications, and help progress your routine safely.

Physical therapists are excellent resources, especially for seniors recovering from injuries, surgeries, or joint replacements. A few sessions of professional instruction when starting resistance band training ensures you pick up safe exercise habits, preventing injury long-term.

Here are important aspects a trainer can help with:

- The correct form for each exercise is strengthening the right muscles and avoiding strain.

- Recommend appropriate band resistance levels and progression.

- Prevent overuse injuries through exercise variety.

- Ensure appropriate pace, range of motion, and breathing.

- Provide modifications for pre-existing conditions like osteoarthritis or osteoporosis.

- Develop well-balanced, effective resistance band routines.

- Keep workouts stimulating through varied exercises.

Even periodic check-ins with a fitness pro can optimize safety as you continue resistance band training independently. They will notice dangerous habits you aren't aware of. Don't hesitate to consult an expert if you're unsure about the proper technique for band exercises. It's a worthwhile investment in your health and safety.

Chapter 11: Water Aerobics for Seniors

Water aerobics, or aqua aerobics or water exercise, is an excellent gentle workout for older adults. This exercise is performed in a pool and takes advantage of the water's natural resistance. In this chapter, you will learn about water aerobics - what it is, why it's so great for seniors, and discover water exercises to improve your fitness and overall health. Water provides a low-impact environment, making aerobic activity accessible for folks of all abilities. It's a refreshing way to stay active.

Why Water Aerobics Is Ideal for Seniors

The buoyancy and natural resistance of water are uniquely suited for senior fitness. Water exercise offers numerous advantages that improve seniors' health, independence, and quality of life, from reducing joint pain to enhancing mobility. Here's a closer look at some of the most significant benefits:

1. **Low-Impact Exercise**

One of the greatest perks of exercising in water is that the body is weightless when submerged. Water's buoyancy offsets about 90 percent of a person's body weight, significantly reducing the impact and compression on joints, bones, and muscles. It substantially decreases the risk of overuse injuries and aggravating conditions like arthritis. Seniors with limited mobility on land can move much more freely in the water. Aquatic exercise allows active movement, minimizing the age-related stiffness, soreness, and pain of high-impact activity.

With aerobic water workouts, there is no hard pavement or ground to pound the legs, knees, ankles, and back. All exercises are performed with soft support underfoot. Jumps, kicks, and other intense emotions are naturally cushioned. The fluid resistance of water prevents sudden starts and stops or direction changes that commonly cause land-based sports injuries. Seniors can achieve an energizing pool workout while avoiding joint degeneration and damage. The low-impact quality helps maintain long-term mobility.

Many studies on aquatic exercise conclude significant reductions in pain and improvements in physical function among adults with arthritis, fibromyalgia, back and neck injuries, and other musculoskeletal conditions without exacerbating symptoms. Water aerobics allows active rehabilitation and a return to cardio fitness in a protected environment for seniors requiring a non-weight-bearing workout due to injury, illness, or surgery. The low-impact nature provides comfortable, accessible exercise for all ages and physical abilities.

2. Built-in Resistance Training

Another major benefit of exercising in water is that the viscosity and drag provide natural resistance for every movement. Pushing, pulling, and moving the limbs through water requires significant muscular effort, thanks to the density of the medium. It allows seniors to strengthen and tone all major muscle groups simply by aerobic water exercises.

No weights, resistance bands, or equipment are necessary to overload the muscles. Common water workout moves like jogging, jumping jacks, kicks, and arm patterns will progressively overload the legs, hips, abs, arms, and chest muscles. Deep water exercise increases the resistance for hardcore strengthening even further.

Aquatic resistance training improves muscle mass and strength for seniors, combating age-related muscle tone and atrophy loss. Stronger muscles equate to greater mobility, stability, bone density, and metabolic rate. It makes daily activities like lifting, reaching, and getting up from chairs more manageable.

Water adds multi-directional resistance so the front, back, and side body musculature all get integrated strengthening. Balanced fitness improves posture and prevents injuries. With aquatic exercise, seniors can simultaneously achieve gentle cardio, flexibility enhancement, balance training, and resistance work in one workout. No fitness center membership is required.

3. Safety and Security

Exercising in water is extremely advantageous for seniors for safety and stability. Water's buoyancy reduces the impact of a slip or fall, making it much less risky for older adults with limited mobility or balance impairments. Should a senior lose balance doing a water exercise, recovery is quick and secure.

The viscosity of water creates a stable environment to catch yourself and regain control of your movements. Water aerobics done properly under instruction prevents falls. However, injury risk is minimal if someone trips or stumbles. Aquatic exercise removes the fear of falling on hard surfaces, allowing for confident mobility.

Deep water exercise performed with a buoyancy belt provides the greatest security. The flotation belt keeps seniors vertically suspended in the water, allowing free and painless limb movements unhindered by impact. Classes often position participants in a circle around the pool perimeter for additional stability.

This setup with flotation devices provides comforting security for new aqua exercise participants. Hand buoys provide additional arm flotation and confidence during swimming motions. Proper supervision and safety measures make water aerobics an extremely safe exercise modality for improving health.

4. Cardiovascular Fitness Gains

While low in joint impact, water aerobics still delivers an excellent cardiovascular workout to improve heart and lung fitness. The water resistance makes movements more challenging, raising exertion levels. When performing water exercises, the muscles must work hard to overcome drag forces, intensifying the effort and elevating the heart rate compared to land exercises. Moving vigorously through water works the cardiorespiratory system without harsh impacts.

Studies show heart rates during water aerobics reach up to 70-80% of the maximum for most individuals, sufficient for building endurance. Splashing the water with vigor also adds intensity. Those with joint issues limiting land activity can push themselves aerobically during aquatic programs. Moreover, water contrasts the body heat sufficiently for active cooling effects.

Water aerobics develops cardiovascular fitness, endurance, efficient breathing, and circulation to enhance seniors' health without orthopedic stress. It provides the perfect medium for active cardio exercise among mature adults and athletes. Water aerobics classes offer an invigorating and safe way for seniors to improve their vitality, heart health, and metabolic function.

Water Aerobics Exercises for Seniors

Here are five foundational water exercises perfect for older adults:

1. Water Walking

Walking in the water engages muscles throughout the body while remaining extremely low impact. To water walk:

1. Move to chest-deep or shoulder-deep water in the pool. Stand tall.

2. Walk forward, striding heel to toe steadily, elevating your heart rate. Swing your arms naturally.

3. Focus on extending each stride as long as it is comfortable, keeping a good upright posture. Allow the water resistance to work the leg muscles harder.

4. Walk briskly for 30 minutes, or interval-train by alternating fast and slower walking.

5. For variation, walk backward or sideways, engaging new stabilizing muscles. You can also add crossovers.

6. Use water dumbbells or floats for added upper-body engagement and resistance during the walks.

Water walking provides gentle cardiovascular training, strengthening endurance. The water resistance tones leg and hip muscles while the buoyancy prevents joint strain.

2. Leg Lifts

Leg lifts tone the thighs and hips through a wide range of motion. To perform water leg lifts:

1. Stand in shoulder-deep water, holding the pool wall or edge for balance. Lessen water depth if needed.

2. Keeping one leg planted firmly, slowly lift the other straight out to the side. Lead with your heel, engaging the outer thigh.

3. Raise your leg as high to the side as flexibility allows. Pause 1 second.

4. Slowly lower your lifted leg, maintaining control.

5. Complete 10-15 controlled lifts on each side. Work up to higher repetitions over time.

6. For added difficulty, point and flex the foot as you lift. Or perform small backward and forward circles during the lift.

7. Make sure the hips and shoulders remain square. Don't let your standing leg bend.

Focusing on lifting the leg high against the water's drag will strengthen and tone the thighs, hips, and core, improving stability for daily mobility.

3. Water Jogging

Water jogging provides an excellent cardiovascular challenge while remaining low-impact. To jog in the water:

1. Move to chest-deep water. Engage your core muscles.

2. Keeping your head stable, quickly drive one knee up toward your chest to "jog" in place.

3. Push the knee up forcefully to recruit your hip flexors against the resistance.

4. Alternate jogging legs continuously at a controlled pace for 5 minutes.

5. Add a complementing arm swing that crosses midline as the alternate legs jog.

6. Rise onto your toes with each knee drive for greater calf burn.

7. Work up to jogging for longer durations or interval training slow and fast cycles.

The water resistance powers up a cardiovascular jogging workout without joint pounding for seniors. Jogging works the whole body and elevates the heart rate.

4. Arm Circles

Arm circles strengthen and mobilize the shoulder joints and upper back muscles. To perform water arm circles:

1. Stand comfortably in shoulder-depth water. Turn your palms downward with elbows straight.

2. Leading with your hands, trace small backward circles with both arms simultaneously.

3. Make 10-15 small circles, reverse direction, and trace 10-15 forward arm circles.

4. Focus on controlling the circles - don't fling your arms with momentum.

5. Gradually increase the size of your arm circles as your shoulder flexibility allows.

6. Add hand paddles or aqua weights to increase the resistance if desired.

The upper back and shoulder muscles must stabilize against the water's drag during arm circles. It improves posture and arm mobility for daily tasks.

5. Water Squats

Squats strengthen the leg and gluteal muscles while increasing hip mobility. To perform water squats:

1. Stand in waist- to chest-deep water with feet slightly wider than shoulder-width. Clasp your hands gently in front of your chest.

2. Initiate the motion from your hips as you bend your knees and lower into a squat.

3. Descend until your upper thighs are parallel to the pool floor if able. Keep your knees behind your toes.

4. Press through your heels to drive yourself back up to standing, fully straightening your legs.

5. Complete 10-15 controlled squats for 1-2 sets.

6. Allow your arms to reach forward to counterbalance or swing them by the sides to increase the challenge.

7. Increase the depth and tempo as your leg strength improves. Take breaks as needed.

The water resistance powers up squats, strengthening the legs, glutes, and core without taxing the knees or back. It enhances stability for daily activities.

Safety Tips for Water Aerobics

Water aerobics offers seniors an extremely beneficial exercise in a low-impact, supportive environment. However, taking precautions to gain the advantages safely is vital. Here are five key tips to help seniors stay safe and comfortable while reaping the fitness benefits of aquatic programs:

1. Stay Properly Hydrated

It may seem counterintuitive since you are already immersed in water during aquatic exercise. However, drinking plenty of hydrating fluids before, during, and after water aerobics sessions is crucial. When exercising in warm water, the body and muscles heat up. Even though surrounded by water, sweat still occurs. This fluid loss from sweating, and increased respiration from cardio activity, make proper hydration essential.

Dehydration symptoms like dizziness, nausea, and lethargy must be avoided. Sip water continuously throughout water aerobics classes. Keep a bottle poolside to drink between exercises frequently. Consuming at least 16 oz. of water 30 minutes before a water workout is recommended. Then, replenish with electrolytes and 20 oz. of water after class. Regularly consuming fluids prevents dehydration, maintains blood volume, and allows muscles to function optimally. Proper hydration helps control body temperature during water exercise.

2. Wear Water Shoes

Proper footwear should be worn during all water aerobics classes to ensure secure footing. Water or aquatic shoes provide traction on pool surfaces and protect feet from abrasion. Built-in arch support helps reduce foot fatigue during rigorous water exercises. Choose water shoes made of quick-drying materials that securely enclose the whole foot. Avoid flip-flops or water socks with slippery plastic soles.

Look for water shoes that:

- Offer multi-directional traction on the pool flooring.

- Snugly fit so they don't slide off during kicks and jumps.

- Provide comfortable arch support and heel cushioning.

- Accommodate custom orthotics if needed.

- Resist chlorine and wet environments with durable materials.

Secure water shoes empower safe, stable footwork during low-impact water exercises seniors love. Proper aquatic footwear prevents slips and improves confidence for active participation.

3. Start Slowly and Build Up Gradually

For those new to water aerobics, starting slowly and gradually increasing duration and intensity is wise. Attempting too vigorous a routine too quickly can lead to next-day soreness, injury, or discouragement. The viscosity of water provides plenty of natural resistance, so no need to overexert. Begin with 10-15 minutes of simple water walking and arm and leg movements to learn ideal pacing.

After a few weeks, as fitness improves, work up to 25-30 minute sessions. Incrementally increase the pace of exercises like water jogging. Add more challenging moves like crossovers or backward walks when ready. Taking time to adapt safely prevents overtraining injuries. Patience in building an aquatic fitness base ensures water aerobics remain fun and rewarding.

It's smart to start conservatively when returning to water aerobics after an injury or extended hiatus. Allow the body to readapt before attempting your prior duration and intensity. Listen closely to your body's signals when ramping up water aerobics routines after a layoff. Soreness taking more than 48 hours to resolve or experiencing sharp joint pains means scaling back and rebuilding more gradually.

4. Listen to Your Body

Pay close attention to how your body feels during water aerobics sessions, and modify exercises accordingly. Aquatic exercise should never cause sharp pain. Lingering discomfort in joints, muscles, or ligaments means an exercise needs adjustment. Communicate openly with the class instructor regarding bothersome movements.

Here are some important signs to heed:

- Joint or muscle pain that persists.

- Wheezing, chest tightness, or breathing difficulty.

- Dizziness, excessive fatigue, or nausea.

- Skin chafing from swimwear.

- Calf cramping or foot soreness.

Minor tweaks like reducing the arm range of motion, lowering water depth, or slowing the kick tempo can prevent issues. Allow modifications until the exercises become comfortable. Listening carefully to your body helps ensure water aerobics remains gentle, safe, and effective.

5. Learn Proper Form from Certified Instructors

Seeking instruction from certified water aerobics teachers is highly recommended for optimal safety. Qualified instructors have the knowledge and experience to teach ideal techniques, provide modifications, and ensure appropriate pacing and precautions. Classes allow new participants to learn proper form, preventing strain. Choose an instructor certified by organizations like the Aquatic Exercise Association. Avoid teachers without accredited training in aquatic exercise.

A quality water aerobics instructor should:

- Hold an accredited certification in water exercise instruction.

- Have substantial experience teaching older adults.

- Offer modifications for different fitness levels.

- Provide feedback on form, pacing, and safety.

- Monitor participants and stop dangerous movements.

- Adjust routines based on attendees' needs and responses.

Proper form prevents injury and improper muscle recruitment. Expert instruction instills safe exercise habits so you can continue benefitting from water aerobics without risk. Investing in professional guidance makes water exercise more rewarding.

Water aerobics is an awesome, super fun way to get fit and feel great overall. As you keep doing these water workouts regularly, you'll get stronger, improve your balance, and make your heart and lungs healthier. Besides the physical benefits, you enjoy the relaxing, refreshing feeling of being in the pool. It's a double win - you get a good workout and float around in the water. So, don't merely think of water aerobics as exercise. It's an activity that can boost your fitness and your entire well-being.

Chapter 12: Mind-Body Practices for Seniors

Keeping your mind and emotions happy and healthy is imperative as you age. Mind-body exercises combining gentle movement with mindfulness and relaxation can holistically boost wellness. In this last chapter, you will learn about fabulous mind-body practices for seniors. These combo workouts provide physical and mental benefits in one harmonious routine. It's a wonderful blend to help seniors stay active and feel content in body and mind.

The Power of Mind-Body Practices

Mind-body practices like yoga, meditation, and tai chi integrate exercise, breathing techniques, and mindfulness to benefit the body and mind. Research shows these practices offer a variety of perks enhancing the health and well-being of older adults, including:

1. Stress Reduction

One of the main advantages of mind-body practices is they help reduce stress. Seniors often deal with major life changes that can be stressful, like retirement, health issues, losing loved ones, and physical decline. This stress impacts mental and physical health, contributing to problems like anxiety, depression, high blood pressure, and a weakened immune system.

Mind-body practices, especially meditation are great stress management tools. Meditation activates the body's relaxation response, which counters the fight-or-flight mode triggered by stress. As stress hormones decrease, the heart rate slows, blood pressure drops, breathing deepens, and muscles relax. Essentially, regular meditation retrains the nervous system to be less reactive to stress. Yoga, tai chi, and deep breathing offer similar stress-busting benefits.

By lowering stress, mind-body practices help improve seniors' overall well-being and ability to take life as it comes. With less anxiety and worry occupying their minds, day-to-day life becomes more pleasant and manageable. Mind-body practices, even for 15-20 minutes daily, give seniors a healthy way to control their stress.

2. Mindfulness

Mind-body practices cultivate mindfulness, maintaining present-moment awareness with openness, curiosity, and acceptance. It means observing thoughts and feelings without judging them.

Being mindful is the opposite of dwelling on the past or worrying about the future, which is common among seniors. Rumination and worry intensify stress and prevent seniors from enjoying the moment.

Mind-body techniques guide seniors into being more present-focused. Meditation develops mindfulness by having seniors tune into sensations, sounds, or breaths. During yoga, seniors enhance mindfulness by moving slowly and deliberately between poses. Tai chi brings mindful awareness to body movements.

Mindfulness strengthens focus, emotional resilience, and mental sharpness. It enhances seniors' capacity to respond to stress thoughtfully rather than being overwhelmed by fears or regrets. Mindfulness allows seniors to gain perspective and appreciate simplicity and everyday joys. By being fully engaged in the present, life becomes richer.

3. Physical Benefits

Many mind-body practices provide physical perks supporting healthy aging. For example, yoga improves balance, strength, and flexibility through practicing seated and standing postures. Moving through the poses with control helps seniors perform daily activities more safely and efficiently. Yoga enhances posture and joint health.

Similarly, the slow, graceful motions of tai chi build core strength, balance, and stability. Often called "meditation in motion," tai chi unites body awareness, breathing, and mental focus. Its movements promote muscle and joint health while improving aerobic fitness.

The physical gains include fewer falls, quicker recovery from illness or injury, and greater independence. As balance, mobility, and vigor improve, seniors feel more self-assured engaging in activities, knowing they have the strength and stability to do so safely.

Mind-body practices incorporating meditation reduce pain perception by helping seniors mentally detach from discomfort. It makes chronic pain more tolerable and less reliant on pain medication.

Mind-body practices enable seniors to enjoy their later years in a strong, fit body. Regular practice allows seniors to maintain and improve their physical abilities well into old age.

4. Pain Management

As noted earlier, mind-body practices can help seniors manage chronic pain. Most seniors deal with persistent pain due to arthritis, nerve damage, surgery, injury, or sickness. Opioids are commonly prescribed for chronic pain, but long-term use carries risks like addiction, constipation, confusion, and increased falls. Mind-body practices provide a safer chronic pain management option.

Meditation and yoga have been shown to decrease pain by lowering stress, relaxing muscles, and increasing pain tolerance. For example, mindfulness meditation teaches seniors to neutrally observe pain sensations, which helps detach them from the unpleasantness. Yoga releases muscle tightness, worsening pain.

Tai chi has proven effective for pain relief in seniors with knee arthritis, providing benefits similar to physical therapy. Its slow, fluid motions improve circulation and relax tense muscles. Simple breathing exercises redirect seniors' attention away from the pain.

Regular mind-body practice allows seniors to actively self-manage pain instead of merely taking medication. They learn skills to alter their pain perception, leading to more independence and control, fewer medication side effects, and improved physical and emotional quality of life.

5. Better Sleep

Lastly, mind-body practices often lead to higher-quality sleep in seniors. Between 40 and 70% of seniors struggle with chronic sleep issues like difficulty falling asleep, staying asleep, and early waking. Poor sleep diminishes hormone balance, metabolism, mood, and thinking skills. Ongoing sleep deprivation jeopardizes seniors' health.

The relaxation response triggered by mind-body practices helps normalize sleep cycles. Yoga and meditation calm the nervous system, slowing breathing, lowering blood pressure, and relaxing muscles to prepare the body for restful sleep. Mindfulness quietens the mind, making it easier to detach from worries that interfere with sleep. Mind-body practices lead to deeper, more restorative sleep.

Tai chi breathing techniques promote relaxation. The low-intensity physical activity of tai chi helps seniors fall asleep more easily at night. However, exercise should be done at least 4 hours before bedtime to prevent sleep disruption.

Quality sleep enhances seniors' well-being. They experience improved energy, mood, cognitive function, and memory. By adopting mind-body practices, seniors give themselves the gift of healthy, rejuvenating sleep.

Mind-Body Practices for Seniors

Mental and physical abilities change with age. Adopting mind-body practices can help seniors navigate these changes gracefully while maintaining health and wellness. Mind-body techniques integrate physical activity, breathing exercises, and mindfulness to benefit the whole person. Here are excellent mind-body practices for seniors:

1. Tai Chi

Tai chi involves slow, flowing bodily movements emphasizing balance, flexibility, and breath control. Of all the mind-body practices, tai chi is especially effective for improving balance and stability in seniors. Loss of balance is common with age and significantly increases the risk of falls and injury.

The controlled stepping and weight shifting in tai chi helps seniors improve their balance skills. The practice strengthens core and leg muscles critical for stability. It enhances mind-body awareness, supporting better coordination and reaction time in avoiding falls. Studies show that tai chi reduces the number and severity of falls in seniors.

The mental focus and deep breathing of tai chi provide stress relief, known to fortify the immune system and cardiovascular health. The meditative nature of the practice creates a calm and inner peace. Tai chi is suitable for all fitness levels and can be done standing or seated. It is a holistic mind-body activity with physical and mental benefits for seniors.

2. Qi Gong

Qi gong is an ancient Chinese mind-body practice comprising gentle movements, breathing techniques, and focused intention. "Qi" refers to the body's life force or energy flow. "Gong" means skill cultivation. So, Qi Gong aims to cultivate skills in optimizing energy flow.

Qi gong's slow, simple movements enhance flexibility, strength, balance, and cardiovascular fitness. Controlled breathing exercises known as "tuna" promote deep relaxation. Qi gong incorporates self-massage and meditation to harmonize the body and mind. Regular practice helps seniors feel energized, flexible, strong, and peaceful.

Qi gong exercises focusing on balance can help seniors reduce their risk of falls. Mental concentration and meditation enhance mind-body connection and awareness. It allows seniors to move through the forms with stability and grace. Qi gong is a wonderful mind-body practice for seniors looking to maintain or restore their physical and mental functioning.

3. Yoga

Yoga is likely one of the most well-known mind-body practices. It originated in India thousands of years ago and has become popular worldwide for people of all ages. Yoga combines physical postures and stretches, breath control techniques, and meditation or mindfulness. The practice aims to unite the mind, body, and spirit.

Yoga improves flexibility, aiding in stability and injury prevention. Moving through postures gently stretches muscles and joints, improving the range of motion. It allows seniors to reach, bend, and turn for household tasks and personal care more easily. Yoga breathing exercises strengthen the diaphragm and lungs. The combined physical postures and breathwork improve circulation, oxygenation, and lung capacity.

Yoga benefits balance as seniors move mindfully from pose to pose. The mental focus required enhances mind-body connection and coordination. There are specialized yoga classes for seniors, like chair yoga, that adapt poses so they can be done comfortably and safely while seated. Yoga boosts physical functioning and provides stress relief and mental clarity. The practice leaves seniors feeling calm, centered, and mentally focused.

4. Meditation

Meditation is a mind-body technique involving quieting the mind and tuning into the present moment. It cultivates mindfulness or purposeful awareness without judgment. Meditation has many styles, but most direct seniors to focus on something specific, like their breathing, a repeated phrase, or a visual object.

A regular meditation practice reduces rumination over past regrets and worries about the future. Staying mindfully present enhances seniors' ability to appreciate and engage with each experience fully. It provides a perspective for inner peace and joy.

Meditation reduces stress hormones and nervous system activity so seniors can sleep, relax, and manage everyday challenges skillfully. By creating a sense of calm, meditation relieves anxiety, depression, and pain perception. Additionally, it slows age-related decline in memory and cognitive skills. Meditation helps seniors preserve their mental acuity well into old age. Only 10 to 20 minutes daily provides benefits.

5. Pilates

Pilates is a mind-body practice that builds core muscle strength, flexibility, and balance. Controlled breathing techniques are essential. Classes involve mat exercises or specialized Pilates equipment.

Pilates enhances stability and posture, reducing the risk of injury from falls. It improves mobility, making moving about freely and engaging in daily activities easier. Pilates boosts mind-body awareness, helping seniors move coordinated and gracefully.

The core strengthening involved benefits seniors in maintaining good posture. A strong core eases back pain and allows seniors to stand tall. Pilates can be adapted for those with physical limitations, but always check with your physician before starting a new exercise program. Pilates provides seniors with strength and stamina benefits without high impact or strain.

6. Deep Breathing Exercises

Deep breathing exercises offer simple mind-body benefits accessible to every senior. Breath techniques can be done anywhere, anytime. They quickly create a physiological shift that promotes relaxation. Deep breathing stimulates the parasympathetic nervous system, reducing heart rate, lowering blood pressure, and relaxing muscle tension.

Seniors can practice taking slow, steady breaths from the diaphragm, focusing on the rise and fall of the abdomen. Slow exhales that are twice as long as the inhales are especially calming. Even 1-2 minutes of deep breathing provides almost immediate stress relief.

Adding visualization can enhance the relaxation effects. As seniors inhale, they can imagine breathing in gratitude, joy, or inner strength. They can visualize breathing out stress, pain, or anxiety as they exhale. This simple mindfulness exercise relieves anxiety and helps seniors feel more energized and optimistic.

Getting Started with Mind-Body Practices

Mind-body practices provide multifaceted benefits, from reducing stress to improving physical functioning. However, getting started with a new mind-body routine can be challenging. Beginners need proper guidance and an approach that sets them up for success. Here are tips to help seniors successfully adopt mind-body techniques:

1. Choose a Practice

The first step is to select one mind-body practice to focus on. Consider which benefits are most appealing and choose accordingly. For example, yoga improves flexibility and reduces pain. Tai chi enhances balance and stability. Meditation relieves anxiety and mental clutter.

It often works best to start with only one practice, allowing you time to learn the techniques properly before adding more. Moreover, it keeps your routine simple and manageable.

2. Find a Class or Instructor

Taking a class is ideal for beginners. An experienced instructor will teach you proper techniques and safety. Classes provide supervision and feedback that prevents injury. The camaraderie of other classmates helps motivate you to attend regularly.

Look for classes specifically designed for seniors that move at an appropriate pace. The instructor should emphasize safety and adapting poses or movements to individuals' ability levels. Don't be shy about informing the instructor if you need additional modifications.

If classes are unavailable, consider private lessons. An instructor can personalize the practice to your needs in a one-on-one setting. Tai chi, Pilates, and yoga studios offer private sessions. Research and ask local communities or social media to find an instructor willing to do home visits.

3. Start Slowly

Never overdo it when starting a new practice. Begin with shorter, basic sessions and build gradually. This approach gives your body time to adjust and prevents pain or injury.

For example, start with 5-10 minutes of gentle yoga or meditation for the first week or two. Then, increase to 15-20 minutes, remaining at an easy intensity. Build slowly from there, listening to your body's signals. Moving too intensely too soon can lead to strained muscles, soreness, and frustration.

4. Stay Consistent

Consistently practicing is fundamental to experiencing benefits. Sporadic practice may provide some relief or fitness gains, but a regular, cumulative practice truly transforms body and mind holistically.

Set a designated time each day or every few days that you devote to practicing. Integrate this into your routine, like brushing your teeth or taking medication. Mark it on your calendar and set reminders if needed. A regular practice schedule will help you stick with it.

5. Practice Mindfulness

Mind-body practices are about more than physical movements. They involve focused awareness and conscious breathing. Be mindfully engaged in each moment with curiosity and presence. Observe how your body feels moving through the forms. Notice thoughts and emotions that arise without judgment.

Tune into the sensory aspects - textures, sounds, sights, and smells around you. This present focus will deepen your practice. Combining physicality, breathwork, and mindfulness makes mind-body practices uniquely beneficial.

6. Modify as Needed

Listen to your body, and don't hesitate to modify it as needed. You may need to adjust your stance, reduce the range of motion, or substitute a different pose or movement. Only do what feels right in the moment.

The instructor should provide alternatives, but don't be afraid to speak up about discomfort or difficulty with aspects of the practice. Your safety and enjoyment come first.

You can use props like cushions, blocks, or chairs to help modify poses or movements to your capability and comfort. Adapt the practice so it works optimally for you.

Conclusion

Stretching is vital as you age to stay active and independent. Seniors can enjoy significant physical and mental perks by making flexibility training a regular habit. This book has guided you to develop a safe, effective stretching routine and the motivation to stick with it.

By now, you know how declining muscle mass and stiff joints limit mobility as you age. However, practicing stretches that target all the major muscle groups can dramatically improve comfort and range of motion. Warming up first to maximize benefits and avoid injury is wise. The step-by-step stretching sequences in this book furnish a complete flexibility workout. Balance exercises further boost stability.

Furthermore, chair stretches make these techniques accessible to anyone. Yoga and Pilates can take flexibility to the next tier. Setting goals, tracking progress, and accountability help make stretching a lifelong habit.

Seniors now have tailored programs and tips to enhance flexibility through stretching. Merely 10 minutes a day delivers results. Improved range of motion equates to better mobility, balance, and independence. All it takes is the commitment to practice regularly and patiently build skills. Hopefully, this book has given you the knowledge and motivation to make stretching a rewarding daily ritual.

References

Aung, M. N., Yuasa, M., Koyanagi, Y., Aung, T. N. N., Moolphate, S., Matsumoto, H., & Yoshioka, T. (2020). Sustainable health promotion for the seniors during COVID-19 outbreak: a lesson from Tokyo. Journal of Infection in Developing Countries, 14(04), 328–331.

Bherer, L., Erickson, K. I., & Liu-Ambrose, T. (2013). A review of the effects of physical activity and exercise on cognitive and brain functions in older adults. Journal of Aging Research, 2013, 1–8.

Cabanas-Valdés, R., Bagur-Calafat, C., Girabent-Farrés, M., Caballero-Gómez, F. M., Hernández-Valiño, M., & Urrútia, G. (2016). The effect of additional core stability exercises on improving dynamic sitting balance and trunk control for subacute stroke patients: a randomized controlled trial. Clinical Rehabilitation, 30(10), 1024–1033.

Chae, B., Kim, K., Hwang, P., Seong, D., Yoonseongdeok, & Duck, P. G. (2017). Effects of Pilates Exercise on senior Fitness Test and Reaction Time of the Elderly. The Korean Society of Sports Science, 26(6), 1169–1179.

Chodzko-Zajko, W., Proctor, D. N., Singh, M. a. F., Minson, C. T., Nigg, C. R., Salem, G. J., & Skinner, J. S. (2009a). Exercise and physical activity for older adults. Medicine and Science in Sports and Exercise, 41(7), 1510–1530.

DiBrezzo, R., Shadden, B. B., Raybon, B. H., & Powers, M. (2005). Exercise Intervention Designed to Improve Strength and Dynamic Balance among Community-Dwelling Older Adults. Journal of Aging and Physical Activity, 13(2), 198–209.

Gergley, J. C. (2013). Acute effect of passive static stretching on Lower-Body strength in moderately trained men. Journal of Strength and Conditioning Research, 27(4), 973–977.

Goodpaster, B. H., Park, S. W., Harris, T. B., Kritchevsky, S. B., Nevitt, M. C., Schwartz, A. V., Simonsick, E. M., Tylavsky, F. A., Visser, M., & Newman, A. B. (2006). The loss of skeletal muscle strength, mass, and quality in Older adults: The Health, Aging and Body Composition Study. The Journals of Gerontology: Series A, 61(10), 1059–1064.

Hinrichs, T., Bucchi, C., Brach, M., Wilm, S., Endres, H. G., Burghaus, I., Trampisch, H., & Platen, P. (2009). Feasibility of a multidimensional home-based exercise programme for the elderly with structured support given by the general practitioner's surgery: Study protocol of a single arm trial preparing an RCT [ISRCTN58562962]. BMC Geriatrics, 9(1).

Kim, K., Han, J. W., & Kim, Y. M. (2019b). Effects of elastic band resistance exercises with breathing techniques on pulmonary function in female seniors. Journal of Exercise Rehabilitation, 15(3), 419–423.

Krucoff, C., Carson, K. M., Peterson, M. J., Shipp, K. M., & Krucoff, M. W. (2010). Teaching yoga to Seniors: Essential considerations to enhance safety and reduce risk in a uniquely vulnerable age group. Journal of Alternative and Complementary Medicine, 16(8), 899–905.

Noradechanunt, C., Worsley, A., & Groeller, H. (2017). Thai Yoga improves physical function and well-being in older adults: A randomised controlled trial. Journal of Science and Medicine in Sport, 20(5), 494–501.

Ouellette, M., LeBrasseur, N. K., Bean, J. F., Phillips, E. M., Stein, J., Frontera, W. R., & Fielding, R. A. (2004). High-Intensity resistance training improves muscle strength, Self-Reported function, and disability in Long-Term Stroke survivors. Stroke, 35(6), 1404–1409.

Sá, M. A., Neto, G. R., Costa, P. B., Gomes, T. M., Bentes, C. M., Brown, A., & Novaes, J. (2015). Acute Effects of Different Stretching Techniques on the Number of Repetitions in a Single Lower Body Resistance Training Session. Journal of Human Kinetics, 45(1), 177–185.

Soonhee, K., Hwang, S., Klein, A. B., & Kim, S. H. (2015b). Multicomponent exercise for physical fitness of community-dwelling elderly women. Journal of Physical Therapy Science, 27(3), 911–915.

Torres, E. M., Kraemer, W. J., Vingren, J. L., Volek, J. S., Hatfield, D. L., Spiering, B. A., Ho, J. Y., Fragala, M. S., Thomas, G. A., Anderson, J. M., Häkkinen, K., & Maresh, C. M. (2008). Effects of Stretching on Upper-Body Muscular Performance. Journal of Strength and Conditioning Research, 22(4), 1279–1285.